A STRATEGIC PLAN FOR EFFECTIVE HEALTH SERVICES

Shailendra Priyadarshi

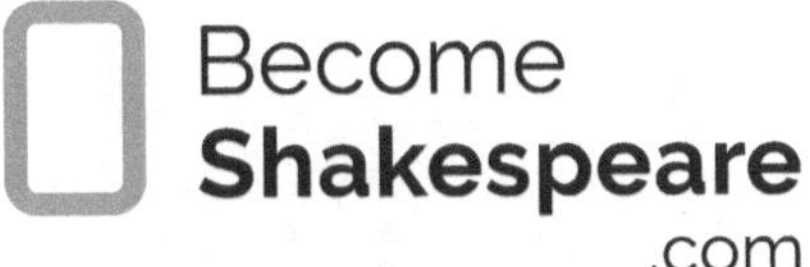

First Published in 2020

Becomeshakespeare.com
One Point Six Technologies Pvt Ltd.
119-123, 1st Floor, Building J2, B - Wing, Wadala Truck Terminal,
Wadala East, Mumbai, Maharashtra, India, 400022.
T: +91 8080226699

Wordit Art Fund helps deserving authors publish their work by providing monetary support. To apply for funding, please visit us at www.BecomeShakespeare.com

ISBN - 978-93-90543-24-3

About the Author

"Dr. Shailendra Priyadarshi has worked in different capacities in both the Government and Private sector with great success providing great service in all the departments he has worked. Starting as a Medical Officer to Chief Medical Officer(Selection Grade), Assistant Commandant to Commandant(Medical) in different organizations he is presently working as a Consultant and Advisor to different companies with outstanding results.He is a B.Sc(Hons.),with MBAs from two institutions of repute(IIBM &JU), besides having an MBBS, and MD(Chest Medicine) with an M.Phil, and Ph. D from BITS_Pilani and associated centers of Excellence.

He has been well guided by a host of extremely talented and revered Scholars/Teachers/Advisors from different fields of study. It is worth mentioning the invaluable contributions of Dr.(Mrs) P.K. Prasad, Mr. S.N. Prasad, Mrs. Aruna Sahay, Mr. S.N. Sahay and family members, Shri Gyan Ranjan, and family members Mr. Sanjeev Sharma, Mr. A.C. Negi, Dr. Nirupama Prakash, Dr. Ravi Prakash, Dr. Neera Dhar, Dr. C.R. Roy, Dr. Chakraborthy, Dr. A.B. Balsara, Dr. J. Tripathy, Dr. S.K. Verma, Mr. Saurabh, and family members, Mr. Praveer and family members, Mrs. Babita, Akshay, and a host of known and unknown dignitaries.

The grace of the Almighty Father, Lord Sai, Queen Mother et al is well emphasized in this work to come to fruition for the benefit of all."

ACKNOWLEDGEMENTS

In any epoch making embellishment the contribution of different elements cannot be over emphasized. It is a natural process of nuts and bolts coming into play in the cogwheel of the sublime task, which is being performed for the benefit of the entire mankind. Similar is the case with the present study–**"A Strategic Plan for Effective Health Services–A Study for Sashastra Seema Bal."**

The contribution of different people, directly or indirectly involved for a successful completion of an endeavor-just can't be overlooked. Anybody becoming one such is definitely bound to perish. Everybody can't be mentioned by name, but they know who and what they are and I thank all of them for their collegiality, counsel and friendship. However, a few of them definitely require mentions that have contributed immensely to the strategic Planning process.

The active support rendered by the Vice Chancellor BITS – Pilani Professor B. N. Jain, DEAN, Academic Research Division, Professor Sanjay Kumar Verma is worth mentioning, who have been providing viable inputs since long.

I am indebted to Dr. C.R.Roy, my guide and teacher during this study that can't be forgotten who despite his busy schedules at North Bengal Medical College & Hospital and the Polyclinic which he is the Director. He gave his valuable time and considered opinion, whenever I have required. Regular interaction was the order of the day.

I can't forget Dr. Y. K. Gupta, I/C Training & Operations, Regional Institute of Health and family Welfare, Jammu for his emphasis upon both man and material for which he himself went along with me to meet different Institutional Heads, National Informatics

Centre and the Secretariat, besides going all the way from Jammu to Gandhinagar to meet Prof. N.S. Gupta, at the Institute of Management & Public Administration.

Prof. N.S. Gupta, of the Institute of Management & Public Administration", Gandhinagar, led me to the fast track of "how to go about the process of data collection and analysis" besides providing other important specifications.

My thanks are meant for Dr. M.P. Gupta, Director, Health Services, Jammu & Kashmir, Shri G.S. Chib, Dy. Director-Planning, Directorate of Health Services, J&K and Shri Onkar Singh Jasrotia from the Statistical Department, Directorate HS, J&K, who provided the statistical data required for the strategic planning process, besides the staff of SSB posted at different places and levels.

I am greatly indebted to Mrs. Kiran Tandon w/o of our Honorable Inspector General at frontier Headquarters SSB, Patna with whom many points have been discussed every now and then not to mention the IG, Shri Daleep Tandon.

Regular discussions with Mrs. Tanushree Baral & Mr. R. Baral, IPS, IG, SSB, MHA, Govt of India &Dr. (Mrs.) Matangi Jha & Mr.S.K.Jha, IPS, IG, Chambal range, M.P took place for the betterment of the project.

I can't forget Shri N.Sinha who has regularly supported me in my different works and would tell me just one thing- "When the going gets tough, the tough get going, you have it in you – Just keep going, you will definitely reach the goal." The constant support of Mrs. Sinha has been a good morale booster.

The able guidance of Shri Ranjit Sinha- minister from Government of Bihar and a very senior congress leader has helped me a lot in the study of the above-cited subject.

Frogs have got a very high protein content and Shri S. K. Gautam, IPS, IG SSB, Force Hqrs. New Delhi was instrumental in getting the assignments completed in time by showing the path of ascertaining facts through the use of absorbing proteins while doing some home work. Thus the concept of Frogs having high protein content came in to being. He has been a guiding light in different walks of life including this write up on **"A Strategic Plan for Effective Health Services – A Study for Sashastra Seema Bal".**

Shri Gyan Ranjan, M.P.Patron-in-chief of SSHRC (Shridi Sai Hospital and Research Centre) words I can't forget and I remember what he had to say – The development of this country rests in the able hands of the youth. If channelised things can become more viable in the future. I have tried to channelise things in that direction where the grace of the Almighty and my different Gurus has been paramount.

I am also thankful to Smt. & Shri A.C.Negi, IPS, ADG, Sikkim Police fort their heartfelt moral support regularly.

My thanks are due to Commandant, Shri Sanjeev Sharma from 22nd Battalion, Ranidanga now in 39th Battalion at Chattisgarh who as a friend always favored my different works.

My sincere thanks are due to my staff posted at 22nd Battalion Ranidanga in West Bengal who helped me during the writing and compilation process of this work. They would say every now and then that we would together get things done. The moral support often accompanying me at odd hours at odd places, one can't forget.

My thanks are due to my elder brother Shri Saurabh Priyadarshi and family members (Mrs.Anjalee & Shreya) as well as my younger brother Shri Praveer Priyadarshi & family members (Mrs. Guddi & Anvita) who have always egged me on to complete the work.

My debt to all my Staff at the SSB, Hospital, especially Shri Rakesh Pal, DFO (Med), Sh. R.K. Kaushik, DFO (Med), ASI (M) Manas Das, Sh. B.B. Prasad, Pharmacist, Sh. Durlav Borah, ASI (Med), Sh. Luv Kush, ASI (Steno), SFA(W/M) Ekta Das, Sh. M.S. Rao, SFA (Med), Sh. Lalan

Baitha, Ct/N/Ordly, Sh. Surinder Singh Chib, Nursing Assistant, Sh. Ritesh, Ct/N/Ordly.

Can I forget the beautiful computing done by Shri S.Ratan Singh, who did the special layout and everything possible to make it a success.

This work has been dedicated to Dr. P.K. Sinha (M.A, M.Ed., and Ph.D.) and Mr. S.N. Prasad (D.C. Finance), my mother and father without whose good wishes and constant support things could have remained static. I am also thankful to Smt. Aruna Sahay , Shri S.N. Sahay, Shri Niraj Sahay & family members who have supported me every time.

The able guidance of Dr. Ravi Prakash Ex- Dean, ARC Division, BITS-Pilani and Dr. (Mrs.) Nirupama Prakash and Dr. S. B. Mishra DAC Member from BITS Pilani, the help rendered by the faculty members of BITS, Pilani, Rajasthan, Indian Institute of Business Management (IIBM), Patna is further acknowledged. I remember the words of the Prakash family a few years back-whether I will be able to do it-and they just said –you have the capacity and you will be able to excel. I am thankful to the faculty at RCD, BITS, Pilani especially the support provided by Dr. Sharad Shrivastava, Shri Dinesh Kumar and Nucleus Members of Academic Research Division (ARD), Ms. Sunita Bansal and Shri Hemant Jhadav and all others at the department known and unknown. I am also indebted to Prof. Asish Kr Das who all have been of great help over the years.

Lastly, the help and constant support by Mrs. Babita Priyadarshi and Akshay Kushagra has also helped me complete this study.

Finally, errors and omissions – if any- I owe them.

It is prudent to mention the excellent backup that has been provided by "BecomeShakespeare.com" and all its team members especially Ms.Pranali Naidu, Mr.Shreyas Prathamshetti, and all involved in the book publication process. Our sincere thanks are hereby acknowledged.

ABSTRACT

Strategic Planning for health Services is a subject of intensive and extensive investigations by academicians as well as management professionals. Different models and measures have been developed during the last few years and a large number of organizations have used them in different situations and contexts. The thesis tries to assess and evaluate these models & measures to capture the different perceptions and perspectives of Health services Strategic management so as to provide a significant learning for researchers and professional managers- a better understanding.

A raging debate is always there as to how important and big the role of Strategic Planning is there for effective management of health services. We propose that strategic management or planning has a very big role in helping SSBHS to be successful in the   role it has been envisaged to play on the borders. We further propose that if Strategic Planning (SP) is developed early at the entry level in SSBHS the health professionals and the health services can effectively meet the challenges and societal requirements on the borders. Thus, they might also contribute to human capital formation. This thesis aims at studying the applications of Strategic Management in health services for SSB and beneficiaries outside the ambit of SSB found from literature and a few studies available relating to the application of Strategic management in health services besides findings of the feedback received from the Purposive Quota Sampling method applied for collecting data .

This study will be helpful in providing feedback about the potential and limitations of each individual to SSBHS and other stakeholders inside and outside the ambit of SSB.

Though the primary attention of the strategic plan is excellence in health care dispensation, there is simply too much evidence that SSB & other Central Paramilitary Forces (CPF) should not and cannot neglect the development of Training and Infrastructure for Health Services.

Emerging trends necessitate new studies and applied research in the field of Health Services. Building healthy and productive health workers requires the active and intentional development of Strategic skills and competencies as normal and integral part of the process of on job training & education. To achieve this balance perspective, the framework provided by Gupta & Gupta is implemented as a frame to provide legitimate information from SSB Personnel & external beneficiaries.

This study would be instrumental in assessing and analyzing the SSBHS and the external beneficiaries so that the policy makers can better meet the future needs of the SSB Personnel and that of the society. Impact of exogenous variables like age, gender, parental upbringing, and family income etc. influences on SSBHS is also analyzed.

The impact of communication on Para Medical staff of SSB is also tested. Individuals communicate for their personal purpose also. The training programmes thus provide the staff to learn newer systems of management and refreshing their earlier knowledge also. Since the PMS are the backbone of any health service it is essential to have a measure of their understanding in communication (UC) and level of responsibility in communication (RC). Communication, being an aspect of Strategic Management for health services as specified by Duncan, Ginter & Swayne (1995) is important for everyday interactions. However, the aspects of measuring the level of UC and RC have not been reported in contemporary literature.

The idea behind our total approach is that the Health Services will grow into what they are capable of becoming, provided we create awareness in them about the goals & objectives and how to go about attaining them and the SSB authorities create proper conditions for that growth of intelligence. This research is aimed at exploring the linkages and relationships between Strategic Planning and its constituent determinants to provide a better working environment for the SSBHS. It is also about formulating the goals and objectives and how to achieve them for developing a competent environment.

The thesis adopts an exploratory type of research design, which aims at obtaining complete and accurate information. There is enough provision for protection against biases and prejudices and even for a-priori perceptions, which help in improving reliability of data. Using purposive quota sampling technique for this exploratory design, instruments collected data from SSB personnel. However a random sampling method was used by conducting open workshops for external beneficiaries outside the ambit of SSB.

A survey was conducted, which comprises of a cross sectional study in relation to the collection of data by deploying questionnaires and structured interventions with many variables to detect patterns of associations. Cross sectional study facilitates examination of relationships between multiple variables. Hypothesis-based research to test the hypotheses of causal relationships between variables was deployed. Such studies require procedures that will reduce bias and increase reliability. This research incorporates numerous hypothesis statements, which are statistically validated. Moreover, in Strategic planning for health Services Situational Analysis in the form of External Environment Analysis, Existing Health Care Analysis, Internal Environment Analysis and Strength, Weakness, Opportunity & Threat Analysis was also carried out to rule out biases-if any. All the above mentioned analysis helped in the formulation of a Frontier (Divisional) Level Strategic Plan for SSBHS.

The Threat, Weakness, Opportunity, Strength Analysis (TWOS) uses five composite scales such as Clinical, Administrative, Finances, Marketing(publicity) & Management to help formulate a Strategic Alternative and Strategic Choice for SSB Health Services. Based on the different parameters the alternatives at the Secretariat (Corporate) level are growth and degeneration. Growth can be either in the form of Diversification or Vertical Integration whereas degeneration can lead to Divestiture and liquidation. As far as Frontier (Divisional) level strategies are concerned growth in the form of Market Share Building and Market Share Holding are the Strategies of Choice.

A sample size of 344 personnel were selected representing different types of SSB Personnel drawn from a variety of socio- economic, cultural and ethnic background. In a similar manner, 110 samples were drawn from beneficiaries outside SSB representing different professional, ethnic, educational disciplines and groups. Data were collected from different areas in the actionable zone of SSB on IndoNepal Border. To ascertain accuracy and consistency, workshop for SSB Personnel along with personal interviews for officers and Administrators were conducted. Descriptive analysis of the data suggests that the targeted sample was appropriate and the various items developed for the performance measures are significant.

The study follows the relational model of Strategic Management or plan process for the development of the SSBHS. It has four stages or groups or processes-**Situational Analysis, Strategic formulation, Strategic implementation and Strategic Control (Duncan, Ginter & Swayne-1992).** To strategically manage or plan an organization related with health services a clear cut understanding of the forces in our current situation, develop from that understanding a plan or strategy that will move the organization towards our vision of the future, develop the functional level programs that will accomplish the strategy and periodically evaluate the success of the strategy or plan and make necessary changes. In reality, these stages are highly interrelated and may be initiated at any given point of time. For example, a Health Care organization finds that action has to be taken before the Strategy has been formalized or before the Situational analysis has been completed or fully understood. Similarly, the process of controlling may create a whole new understanding of the competition and thus a new strategy.

Situational Analysis consists of investigating the External environment to extract key forces determining external factors. It also analyses the Internal Strengths and weaknesses of the organization besides evaluating the organizations purpose, vision, mission and objective. The organizational strategy must take advantage of opportunities in the environment, avoid external threats, capitalize on internal strengths and reduce the organizations weakness. During the SSBHS plan process the organizations values & culture was also assessed so that a clear understanding of purpose and mission is ascertained.

The next stage is Strategy Formulation. Based on the results of Situational Analysis, the Organizational Goals or Objectives are established, the strategic alternatives are generated and evaluation of the same is done, a strategy determined and a plan of action developed. Based on the organizational setting the formulation stage determines the course of action for the SSBHS. Thus the basics of Strategic Planning depends upon Situational analysis & strategy Formulation. The above studies are presented in the forms of Exhibits and flow charts at different places in a series of events mutually related with each other.

Different statements were tested, which included statements for age, gender and the Socio- economic background of the SSB personnel. The analysis revealed the association and the strength of association of each of the factors. The correlation with communication ability was low but it significantly rose with better qualified SSB personnel.

The research concludes that the plan process for SSBHS is the aggregate of the characteristics and the knowledge and skills that individuals acquire and develop throughout their tenure in SSB. There is undoubtedly evidence-identifying Strategic Management or Plan for SSB health Services as important in predicting personal and Health services success which has a potential implication for the overall success of the policy decisions taken at the centre for the benefit of the CPFs and the society where the SSB is deployed.. However, researchers need to be more cautious in making claims until more evidences are available from the Strategic plan process of different CPFs.

The study highlights ways that are personally meaningful, as well as constructive and meaningful for society. Education, training, and counseling approaches aimed at developing personal excellence in individuals will provide a widely applicable model for making the world a better place. Even though the primary attention of education is academic performance, there is simply too much convincing evidence that SSB and other CPFs should not and cannot neglect the development of goals and objectives for the better management of the health services.. Emerging trends necessitate new studies and applied research on the contributions of the SSB Personnel for having a better health service provider through the SSB health services. . Building healthy and productive SSB employees requires the active and intentional development of the Strategic Plan of SSBHS and its related competencies. Thus the final purpose of the research is to create a platform that can practically be utilized to implement the Goals and objectives envisaged for SSBHS for not only SSB but all the CPFs for the benefit of the Indian people.

Table of Contents

List of Figures

List of Exhibits

List of Table

Chapter 1
INTRODUCTION

1.1 INTRODUCTION:

The chapter introduces SSB or Sashastra Seema Bal, the importance of Effective Health Service, importance of Health Services as a field of Study and presents the background, rationale, significance, objectives, scope, Identifying Burning Issues faced by SSBHS and methodologies adopted to undertake the research. Emergency management and contingency planning are vital for any organization that wants to survive and prosper. Contingency planning can be a time- consuming, costly process and, consequently, it is used in public and private sector entities to varying degrees. In the absence of proper planning, a crisis or disaster could devastate an organization, its people and its assets. As such Strategic Panning will improve the odds of SSB surviving as an organization. "Strategic planning is the process of formulating and implementing decisions about an organization's future direction. This process is vital to every organization's survival because it is the process by which the organization adapts to its ever-changing environment, and the process is applicable to all management levels and all types of organizations" (Kerzner, 2001, p. 15).

SSB or Sashastra Seema Bal came in to existence in the year **1962-63**. SSB was known as ***Special Service Bureau*** at that time and was a department under the **Cabinet Secretariat, Prime Minister's Office, and Government of India.**

The role of the erstwhile Special Service Bureau changed to a **Para Military Force** in the year **2000-   01** after **a group of Ministerial recommendations that Special Service Bureau be converted into a Border Guarding Force**. As such the name of Special Service Bureau was rechristened as Sashastra Seema Bal (SSB) and was placed under the **Ministry of Home Affairs, Government of India as a Central Para Military Force (CPMF)**. Now SSB is a Border Guarding Force (BGF) and is deployed on the **Indo Nepal Border (INB)** as well as **Indo Bhutan Border(IBB)**.

Consequent of its deployment on the Indo Nepal Border as well as Indo Bhutan Border later on- has led to a paradigm shift in the thinking of the force related with its Medical setup.

During the Special Service Bureau days the basic thrust of the Medical set up was in J & K, Rajasthan, Gujarat and North Eastern states like Manipur, Nagaland, Arunachal Pradesh, Assam, etc. However, once SSB shifted to Indo Nepal Border the thrust of the Medical set up of SSB also shifted to states like Sikkim, West Bengal, Bihar, and Utter Pradesh & Uttarkhand whereas on the Indo Bhutan Border the thrust shifted to Bordering districts of Assam, parts of West Bengal and parts of Arunachal Pradesh.

1.2 OBJECTIVES:

The objectives of the study involving the health Services of SSB was related with how to make it effective and efficient in the changing scenario and the day to day challenges that are being faced by the force.

As such the following fields were critically examined-

i   Prevention and control of communicable disease

ii   Effective control and management of HIV/AIDS through VCCT centers,

iii   Effective control and management of Malaria, Kalazar and water borne disease like diarrhea and dysentery,

iv   Rehabilitation programme for the physically handicapped people,

v   Man power development,

vi   Infrastructure development,

vii   Organizational structure – Reconstruction there of,

viii   Economics involvement - Fresh initiatives,

ix   Overweight and Obesity-an overriding problem in SSB,

x   Drug Trafficking & Drug Deaddiction,

xi   Emergency management,

xii   Business continuity,

xiii   Strategic Planning

xiv   Scenario Futuring and

xv   Service to Mankind through WARB (Welfare and Rehabilitation Board).

These fields were analyzed with a goal of developing an integrated strategic contingency planning model for SSB Health Services. This model would assist the organization in bringing their contingency planning program to a strategic level. Contingency planning can be fully integrated with day-to-day business processes if a new mindset is developed after training in the organization. Contingency planning no longer needs to be an isolated, specialized process; rather it should be integrated into the foundation of an organization. An organization is normally in business to stay in business, so practicing contingency planning is a logical component of a successful business operations. Not-for-profit and public sector entities also need to prepare for continuity of services in order to assist constituents and citizens. By including the continuity strategies in the company's strategic plan, they are naturally reviewed periodically and updated when the strategies of the company change.

The business continuity strategies become part of the corporate culture and a natural part of management thinking. Additionally, since this new element is added to the company's existing planning program, the marginal cost associated with maintaining it is substantially reduced. (Stagl, 2003, p.39).

This research puts forth an effort to synthesize and integrate some of the major findings of the studies carried out on SSB Health Services, as they relate to the goals of education and human development. The main goal of these studies was to provide a coherent and practical approach to health services that SSB personnel can learn and apply to stay healthy both physically and mentally, think of career progression, and enhance individual and collective productivity. As such the following goals/objectives were considered in detail during the study for effective health services for Sashastra Seema Bal:

> **Goal1** : **Quality Health Care and Infrastructure Development.**

> **Goal2** : **Health Promotion and protection, prevention of disease and Prepare for any contingency/Emergency.**

> **Goal3** : **Service to Mankind through WARB (Welfare and Rehabilitation Board).**

> **Goal4** : **Research and development with increasing management practices.**

However, despite the large amount of rhetoric on this highly ideological issue there is surprisingly little resource to form a policy or for that matter inform policy makers. The present study tried to examine all the above and other related matters in detail so as to provide a Strategic Plan for effective health services for Sashastra SeemaBal.

1.3 APPROACH/METHODOLOGY:

The approach used in this study was to provide a background in contingency planning processes and then show how strategic planning processes can be applied to make a more effective contingency planning program. Chapter 2 presents the structure of how the evolution of SSB took place over the years. Chapter 3 presents a review of literature in the emergency planning, business continuity, strategic planning and scenario futuring fields besides preventive and social aspects of preventive medicine to provide a foundation for the study. Chapter 4 presents the methodology comprising the Questionnaire method, & Situational analysis comprising the External Environment Analysis, The Existing Health care System, The Internal Environment Analysis. Chapter 5 presents Results & Discussion based on the **Questionnaire & Situational Analysis** in the form of **Inferences (based on the questionnaire)** & **Vision, Mission, Strategic Alternatives & Strategic choice for SSBHS (based on Situational Analysis)**.Chapter6 presents Conclusions in the form of The Frontier (Divisional) level Strategic plan along with recommendations for the benefit of the SSBHS.

The objectives outlined earlier are achieved through the accomplishment of the following tasks:

a) A review of literature related to SSBHS with thematic representation of the phases of development of SSBHS.

b) Development of a theoretical framework based on review of literature and identifying Questionnaires for developing a Strategic Plan for SSBHS.

c) Design and develop vision and mission statements. A review of literature revealed that a number of methods for developing a strategic plan are in use. However, the following six steps appear common to the various approaches:

    i.   Develop vision and mission statements.

    ii.   Create a strategic model.

    iii.   Perform an audit of the organization.

    iv.   Do a gap analysis.

    v.   Complete action plans.

    vi.   Implement theplans.

In other words a Situational Analysis was done which is the *analytical process for any strategy formulation which* included the following-

A.   The External Environment Analysis.

(A-i) The Existing Health Care Systems.

B.   The Internal Environment Analysis.

C.   The Development of the Organization.

    The development of the organization depends upon- Purpose, Vision, Mission and Objectives.

D.   Develop a Strategic Alternative & Strategic Choice. To develop a Strategic Alternative & Strategic Choice for SSB Health Services, especially at the Frontier Level, one has to consider the following aspects in detail:

1.   The hierarchy of SSB organization. (Discussed in Chapter-2)

2.   The TOWS Matrix for evaluating Strategic Alternatives and Strategic Choice.

3.   The Strategic Alternatives at the Frontier Level.

The Strategic Alternatives are further divided into: (i) Corporate Strategies. (ii) Divisional Strategies. (iii) Functional Strategies.

Since, we are concerned with Divisional Level Strategies; hence we will confine ourselves to its formation and selection only.

E.   **The development of the frontier level Strategic Plan.**

A comparative study of responses of SSB Personnel and responses of external beneficiaries outside the ambit of SSB was also considered and studied to finally conclude the development of the frontier level Strategic Plan.

F.   Conclusion &Recommendations.

1.4 LIMITATIONS:

The health system in the changing scenario of SSB faces unparalleled challenges in responding to the increasing complexity of health care. Health system that were capable of providing basic care to population where disease were either simple or complex but self-limiting confront a fatal struggle to keep up with the increasing opportunity that modern science has provided. The challenges are especially vast in under developed countries because the whole world at large is not willing to see millions of people die from treatable disease like Diarrhea, Dysentery, Typhoid, Malaria or Tuberculosis. The community at large through the initiative of Government of India under Ministry of Health and Family Welfare, Ministry of Home through organizations like SSB tries to prolong life for patients suffering from HIV/AIDS. Voluntary Confidential Counseling and Testing (VCCT) centers have been opened in the different units of SSB Medical set up to look into this matter. As a consequence, resources like pharmaceuticals are being provided to patients who are in need of them, but still the required benefits are not percolating down the line, down the rank and file.

This study does not address the information technology (IT) aspects of the Health services due to the complexity and emerging nature of information systems products. IT departments may have very detailed plans in place to recover hardware, software, telecommunication and other systems even in the field of health services planning. These preparations are usually known as *disaster recovery plans*. It is incumbent upon the SSB administration, however, to ensure that their IT departments are fully aware of critical systems and recovery priorities. The three-pronged approach of emergency management, business continuity and disaster recovery, recovery of an organizational can be severely curtailed.

This study also does not specifically address the security of the SSBHS in the organization. Security and contingency planning often go hand-in-hand in organizations. Many security features such as fences, controlled access systems, cameras, etc. are taken into consideration when doing contingency planning. This security field, because of its complexities technically, is beyond the scope of the present study involving the SSB Health services.

Para Medical Staff through the wide-ranging training mechanism should also upgrade in financial management since increasing funds are being made available for purchase of pharmaceutical goods. This study does not include this aspect of development of the contingency planning for SSB Health Services.

1.5 KEY TERMS DEFINED:

To have a functional idea what strategic plan deals with and how it is useful in formulating the strategy for any department one should have a working knowledge about (a) Strategy, (b) Strategic

Planning and related terminology which has been defined as follows:

A. **Strategy**: A strategy is a future oriented plan that provides decision-making guidelines for managers. In a larger senses strategy may be thought as "a pattern that emerges in a stream of decisions regarding the organization about what it wants to do, what it can do and how it should do."

Strategy is about positioning an organization for sustainable competitive advantage. It involves making choices about which industries to participate in, what products and services to offer, and how to allocate corporate resources. Its primary goal is to create value for shareholders and other stakeholders by providing customer value. (de Kluyver and Pearce, 2003, p. 1)

B. **Strategic Planning**: Strategic planning can be defined as the organizational process for identifying the desired future and developing decision guidelines. As such, the result of the strategic planning process is a plan or strategy.

The process by which the guiding members of an organization envision its future and develop the necessary procedures and operations to achieve that future. (Goodstein, Nolan & Pfeiffer, 1993, p. viii)

N.B. : Strategic planning is sometimes used interchangeably with the Strategic Management Process. As such Strategic Management (2) is an externally oriented philosophy of managing an organization that links strategic planning to operational environment (Political, Regulatory, Economic, Technological, Social and Competitive resources, marketing, information system).

C. ***Business Continuity Management Program***: An ongoing management and governance process supported by senior management and resourced to ensure that the necessary steps are taken to identify the impact of potential losses, maintain viable recovery strategies and plans, and ensure continuity of products/services through exercising, rehearsal, testing, training, maintenance and assurance. (DRJ Editorial Advisory Board,2005)

D. ***Business Continuity Team***: Designated individuals responsible for developing, execution, rehearsals, and maintenance of the business continuity plan, including the processes and procedures. Similar terms: disaster recovery team, business recovery team, recovery team. Associated term: crisis response team. (DRJ Editorial Advisory Board,2005)

E. ***Business Impact Analysis (BIA)***: The Business Impact Analysis is a process designed to identify critical business functions and workflow, determine the qualitative and quantitative impacts of a disruption, and to prioritize and establish recovery time objectives. Similar terms: Business Exposure Assessment, Risk Analysis. (DRJ Editorial Advisory Board,2005)

F. ***Crisis Management***: The overall coordination of an organization's response to a crisis, in an effective, timely manner, with the goal of avoiding or minimizing damage to the organization's profitability, reputation, or ability to operate. (DRJ Editorial Advisory Board,2005)

G. ***Crisis Management Team***: A crisis management team will consist of key executives as well   as key role players (i.e. media representative, legal counsel, facilities manager, disaster recovery coordinator, etc.) and the appropriate business owners of critical organization functions. (DRJ Editorial Advisory Board,2005)

H. ***Damage Assessment***: An appraisal or determination of the effects of the disaster on human, physical, economic, and natural resources. (NFPA, 2004, Section 3.3.2, p.1600-4)

I. ***Disaster***: A sudden, unplanned calamitous event causing great damage or loss as defined or determined by a risk assessment and business impact analysis; 1) Any event that creates an inability on an organizations part to provide critical business functions for some predetermined period of time. 2) In the business environment, any event that creates an inability on an organization's part to provide the critical business functions for some predetermined period of time. 3) The period when company management decides to divert from normal production responses and exercises its disaster recovery plan. Typically signifies the beginning of a move from a primary to an alternate location. Similar terms: Business Interruption; Outage; Catastrophe. (DRJ Editorial Advisory Board, 2005)

J. ***Disaster/Emergency Management Program***: A program that implements the mission, vision, and strategic goals and objectives as well as the management framework of the program and organization. (NFPA, 2004, Section 3.3.3, p.1600-4)

K. ***Disaster Recovery Planning***: The technological aspect of business continuity planning. The advance planning and preparations that are necessary to minimize loss and ensure continuity of the critical business functions of an organization in the event of disaster. Similar terms: Contingency Planning; Business Resumption Planning; Corporate Contingency Planning; Business Interruption

Planning; Disaster Preparedness. (DRJ Editorial Advisory Board, 2005)

L. ***Emergency***: An unexpected actual or impending situation that may cause injury, loss of life, destruction of property or cause the interference, loss or disruption of an organization's normal business operations to such an extent that it poses a threat.(DRJ Editorial Advisory Board, 2005)

M. ***Emergency Management/Emergency Planning***: "When disasters threaten or strike a jurisdiction, people expect elected leaders to take immediate action to deal with the problem. The government is expected to marshal its resources, channel the efforts of voluntary agencies and private enterprise in the community, and solicit assistance from outside the jurisdiction if necessary. In all states and most localities, that popular expectation is given force by statute or ordinance. Governments can discharge their emergency management responsibilities by taking four interrelated actions: mitigation, preparedness, response, and recovery. A systematic approach is to treat each action as one phase of a comprehensive process, with each phase building on the accomplishments of the preceding one. The overall goal is to minimize the impact caused by an emergency in the jurisdiction." (FEMA, 1996, p.12)

Five Phases of Emergency Management:

1. Prevention (proposed language): Activities taken to avoid or to stop a disaster/emergency from occurring.

2. Preparedness (Section 3.3.9): Activities, programs, and systems developed and implemented prior to a disaster/ emergency that are used to support and enhance

mitigation of, response to, and recovery from disasters/ emergencies.

3. Response (Section 3.3.11): In disaster/emergency management applications, activities designed to address the immediate and short-term effects of the disaster/ emergency.

4. Recovery (Section 3.3.10): Activities and programs designed to return conditions to a level that is acceptable to the entity.

5. Mitigation (Section 3.3.7): Activities taken to eliminate or reduce the probability of the event, or reduce its severity or consequences, either prior to or following a disaster/ emergency.

(NFPA, 2004, p.1600-4)

N. **Gap Analysis**: A survey whose aim is to identify the differences between BCM/Crisis Management requirements (what the business says it needs at time of an event and what is in place and/or available. (DRJ Editorial Advisory Board,2005)

O. **Hazard**: A natural, technological or social phenomenon that threatens human lives, livelihoods, land use, property or activities. Some hazards may result in a single disaster impact, others are recurrent on a regular (i.e., seasonal) or irregular (random) cycle. The majority are recurrent rather than unrepeatable events. Many types of hazard impact can be characterized by a magnitude-frequency relationship in which the larger the impact the lower its frequency of occurrence. (Alexander, 2002, p.312)

P. **Hazard or Threat Identification**: The process of identifying situations or conditions that have the potential to cause injury to people, damage to property, or damage to the environment. (DRJ Editorial Advisory Board,2005)

Q. ***Incident***: An event, series of events, or set of circumstances that interrupts normal operating procedures and has the potential to precipitate an emergency or crisis. (Gillis, 1996, p. 4)

R. ***Incident Response***: The response of an organization to a disaster or other significant event that may significantly impact the organization, its people, or its ability to function productively. An incident response may include evacuation of a facility, initiating a disaster recovery plan, performing damage assessment, and any other measures necessary to bring an organization to a more stable status. (DRJ Editorial Advisory Board,2005)

S. ***Mission-Critical Application***: An application that is essential to the organization's ability to perform necessary business functions. Loss of the mission-critical application would have a negative impact on the business, as well as legal or regulatory impacts. (DRJ Editorial Advisory Board,2005)

T. ***Operational Risk***: The risk of loss resulting from inadequate or failed procedures and controls. This includes loss from events related to technology and infrastructure, failure, business interruptions, staff related problems, and from external events such as regulatory changes. (DRJ Editorial Advisory Board,2005)

U. ***Risk Assessment/Analysis***: Process of identifying the risks to an organization, assessing the critical functions necessary for an organization to continue business operations, defining the controls in place to reduce organization exposure and evaluating the cost for such controls. Risk analysis often involves an evaluation of the probabilities of a particular event. (DRJ Editorial Advisory Board, 2005)

V.   **Risk Categories**: Risks of similar types are grouped together under key headings, otherwise known as 'risk categories'. These categories include reputation, strategy, financial, investments, operational infrastructure, business, regulatory compliance, outsourcing, people, technology and knowledge. (DRJ Editorial Advisory Board,2005)

W.   **Risk Mitigation**: Implementation of measures to deter specific threats to the continuity of business operations, and/or respond to any occurrence of such threats in a timely and appropriate manner. (DRJ Editorial Advisory Board,2005)

X.   **Scenario**: A pre-defined set of Business Continuity events and conditions that describe, for planning purposes, an interruption, disruption, or loss related to some aspect(s) of an organization's business operations to support conducting a BIA, developing a continuity strategy, and developing continuity and exercise plans. Note: Scenarios are neither predictions nor forecasts. (DRJ Editorial Advisory Board,2005)

Y.   **Stakeholder**: Although there are several ways to classify stakeholders, the most common method is as follows:

Financial Stakeholders

   Stockholders

   Financial institutions (suppliers of capital) Creditors

   The Product/Market Stakeholders

Primary customers Primary suppliers Competitors Unions

> Government agencies

> Local government committees

Organizational Stakeholders

> Executive officers

> Board of Directors

> Employees in general

> Managers

> (Kerzner, 2001, p. 5)

Z.   **System**: A set or arrangement of things so related or connected as to form a unity or organic whole. (Neufeldt, 1994, p.1359)

(Z-i) Workaround Procedures: Interim procedures that may be used by a business unit to enable it to continue to perform its critical functions during temporary unavailability of specific application systems, electronic or hard copy data, voice or data communication systems, specialized equipment, office facilities, personnel, or external services. (DRJ Editorial Advisory Board, 2005)

Chapter 2
STRUCTURING THE EVOLUTION OF SSB

2.1 INTRODUCTION:

SSB or Sashastra Seema Bal came in to existence in the year **1962-63**. SSB was known as *Special Service Bureau* at that time and was a department under the **Cabinet Secretariat, Prime Minister's Office, and Government of India.**

The role of the erstwhile Special Service Bureau changed to a **Para Military Force** in the year **2000-01** after **a group of Ministerial recommendations that Special Service Bureau be converted into a Border Guarding Force.** As such the name of Special Service Bureau was rechristened as Sashastra Seema Bal (SSB) and was placed under the **Ministry of Home Affairs, Government of India as a Central Para Military Force (CPMF).** Now SSB is a Border Guarding Force (BGF) and is deployed on the **Indo Nepal Border (INB)** as well as **Indo Bhutan Border (IBB).**

2.2 EVOLUTION OF SSB:

2.2.1 First phase (1963 – 2000) Theme: Development of SSB

SSB or Sashastra Seema Bal came in to existence in the year **1962-63**. SSB was known as *Special Service Bureau* at that time and was a department under the **Cabinet Secretariat, Prime Minister's Office, and Government of India.**

2.2.2 Second phase (2001 – 2010 & further) Theme: Expansion of SSB on INB

The role of the erstwhile Special Service Bureau changed to a **Para Military Force** in the year **2000-01** after **a group of Ministerial recommendations that Special Service Bureau be converted into a Border Guarding Force**. As such the name of Special Service Bureau was rechristened as Sashastra Seema Bal (SSB) and was placed under the **Ministry of Home Affairs, Government of India as a Central Para Military Force (CPMF)**. Now SSB is a Border Guarding Force (BGF) and is deployed on the **Indo Nepal Border (INB)** as well as **Indo Bhutan Border (IBB)**.

During the expansion phase of SSB issues related with the following were developed-**(1) Manpower development. 2) Organizational structure – Reconstruction thereof. (3) Infrastructure development. (4) Economics involvement-Fresh initiatives.**

1) **Manpower development:**

Specific attempts have been made to develop manpower and streamline the things and make it a smooth operator but still there are road blocks which require sectarian changes and hence it is up to the Sector heads, Bn. heads and Area heads to augment the development of manpower (50,51).

A guiding light is always there who takes care of the things being faced by all and sundry but it is the person at the helm of that unit who requires to put extra effort and motivate heads of unit to implement the schemes for the betterment of the department.

A sector wise distribution of staff under Frontier Hqr. SSB, Patna is as under:

SECTOR HQS WISE STAFF POSITION OF MEDICAL/PARA MEDICAL STAFF UNDER FRONTIER HQR SSB, PATNA.

1.   **(a) MEDICAL OFFICERS UNDER SECTOR HQ. SSB, MUZAFFARPUR:**

SL. NO.	Name of Post	Authorized Strength	Posted strength	Vacant	Surplus	Remarks
01.	MEDICAL OFFICER	11	4	7	--	9thBn. – 1 12thBn.-1 13thBn. -0 14thBn. -2 SHQ. MZP -0 Total-4

(b) PARA MEDICAL STAFFS UNDER SHQ. MUZAFFARPUR:

Sl. No.	Name of post	Authorized Strength	Posted Strength	Vacant	Surplus	Remarks
01.	SI(M)	5	--	5	--	
02.	ASI(M)	5	3	2	--	
03.	HC(M)	12	6	6	-	
04.	CT(M)	5	4	1	-	
05.	CT/N/Ordly	5	4	1	-	
06.	Pharmacy	5	5	-	-	
07.	Lab. Tech	5	2	3	-	
Total		42	24	18	-	

2. (a) MEDICAL OFFICERS UNDER SECTOR HQ. SSB, PURNEA:

SL. NO.	Name of Post	Authorized Strength	Posted strength	Vacant	Surplus	Remarks
01.	MEDICAL OFFICER	9	6	3	--	18[th]Bn. – 1 19[th]Bn.-2 36[th]Bn. -1 28[th]Bn. -0 SHQ. PRN -2 Total - 6

(b) PARA MEDICAL STAFFS UNDER SHQ. PURNEA:

Sl. No.	Name of post	Authorized Strength	Posted Strength	Vacant	Surplus	Remark
01.	SI(M)	3	-	3	--	
02.	ASI(M)	4	2	2	--	
03.	HC(M)	10	7	3	-	
04.	CT(M)	4	4	-	-	
05.	CT/N/Ordly	4	3	1	-	
06.	Pharmacy	-	-	-	-	
07.	Lab. Tech	-	-	-	-	
Total		25	16	9	-	

3.   **(a) MEDICAL OFFICERS UNDER SECTOR HQ. SSB, RANIDANGA:**

SL. NO.	Name of Post	Authorized Strength	Posted strength	Vacant	Surplus	Remarks
01.	MEDICAL OFFICER	7	5	2	--	22^{nd}Bn. – 2 24^{th}Bn.-2 21^{th}Bn. -1 29^{th}Bn. -0 SHQ. RDA -1 Total - 6

(b) PARA MEDICAL STAFFS UNDER SHQ. RANIDANGA:

Sl. No.	Name of post	Authorized Strength	Posted Strength	Vacant	Surplus	Remarks
01.	SI(M)	2	-	-	-	
02.	ASI(M)	3	2	1	--	
03.	HC(M)	7	6	1	-	
04.	CT(M)	3	2	1	-	
05.	CT/N/Ordly	4	3	1	-	
06.	Pharmacy	3	3	-	-	
07.	Lab. Tech	4	3	1	-	
Total		26	19	5	-	

SUMMARY:

UNDER SHQ. MZP	:	AS	PS	V	S
MEDICAL		**11**	**4**	7	0
PARAMEDICAL		42	24	18	0
		53	28	25	0
UNDER SHQ. PRN		AS	PS	V	S
MEDICAL		9	6	3	0
PARAMEDICAL		25	16	9	0
		34	22	12	0
UNDER SHQ. RDA		AS	PS	V	S
MEDICAL		7	5	2	0
PARAMEDICAL		26	19	5	0
		33	24	7	0
GRAND TOTAL :	:	**120**	**74**	**44**	**0**

2) **Organizational structure – Reconstruction thereof.**

In the present setup the following graphic depiction gives a pen picture of the organizational setup (53) where at the helm of affairs HonorableHer Excellency The President of India presides.

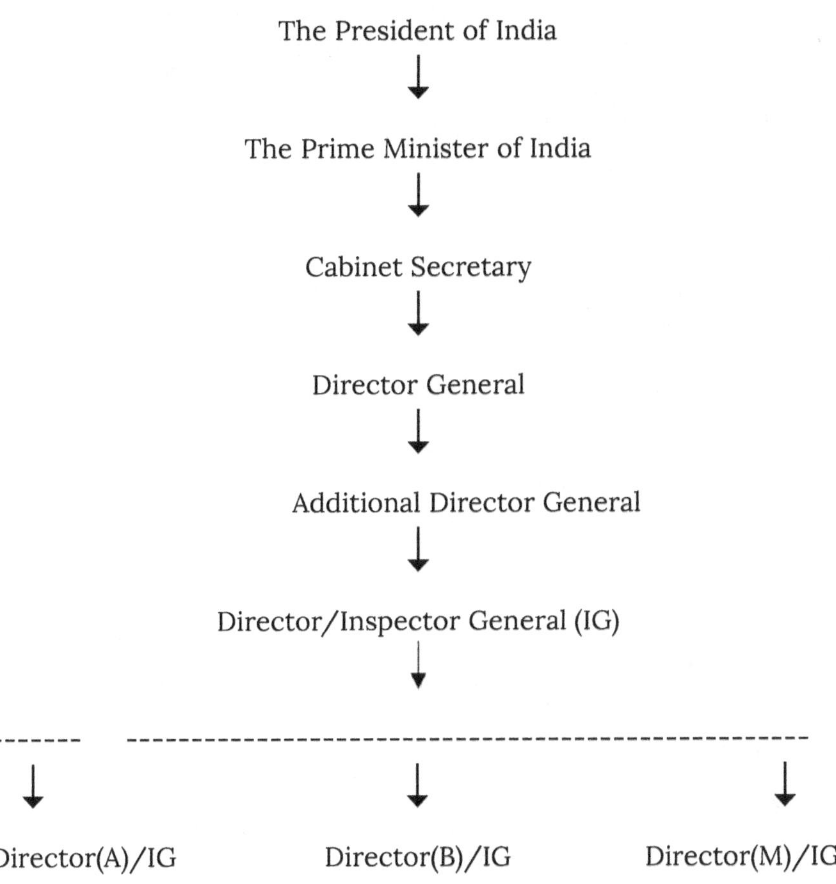

FRONTIER LEVEL

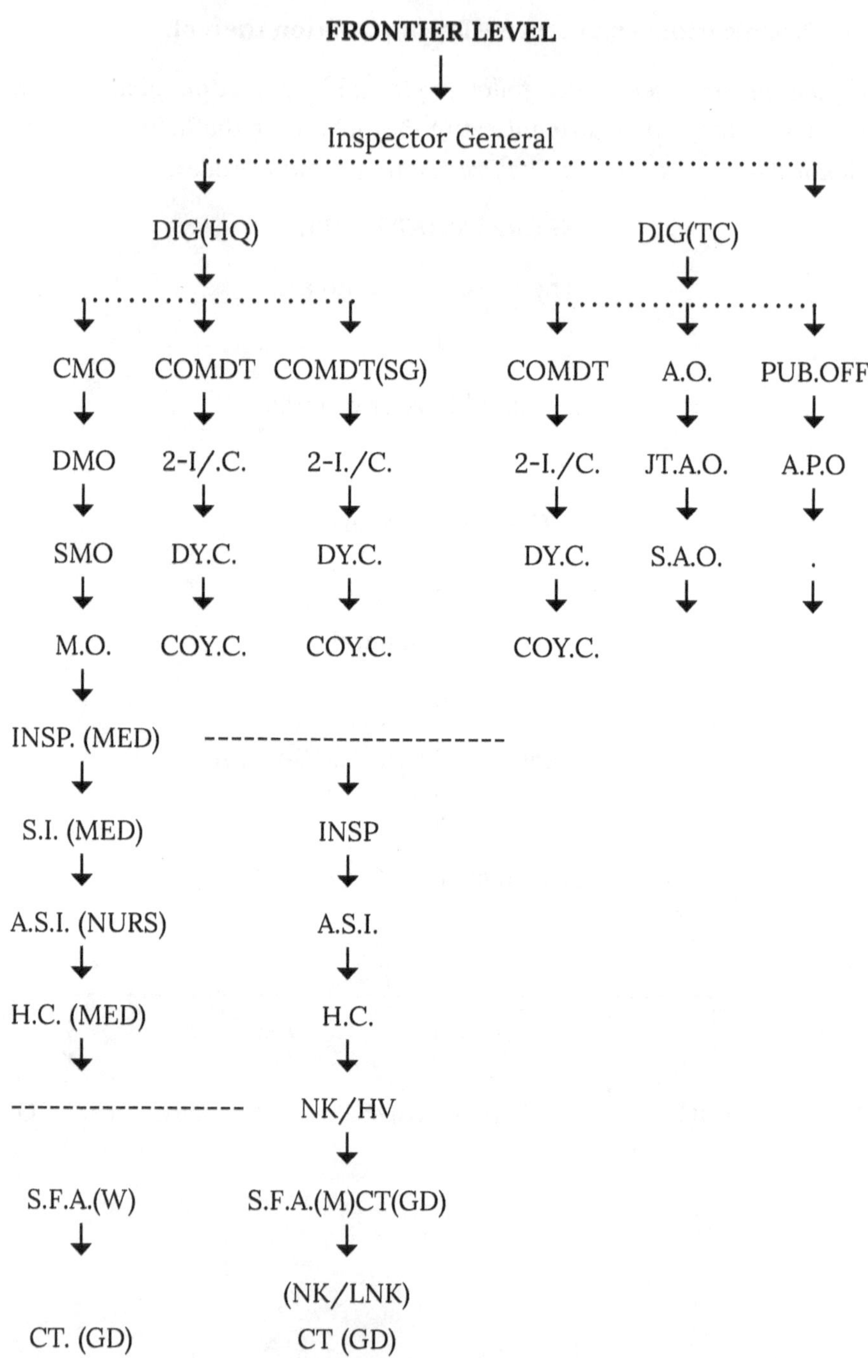

FUNCTIONAL LEVEL

↓

Area Organizer

↓

JT. A.O.

↓

S.A.O.

↓

C.O.

↓

D.F.O. (MED)

↓

A.F.O. (MED)

↓

S.F.A. (MED)

At the Frontier level the Departments have been divided as follows:

Frontier Level:

i.	Group Centre/Bn	iv.	Vet. Services
ii.	Training Centre	v.	Publicity & Marketing Dep't.
iii.	Medical Services	vi.	Women's Area Training School

Medical Services:

Concentrating on the Medical Services, it is proposed to reorient the organizational structure in the following manner:

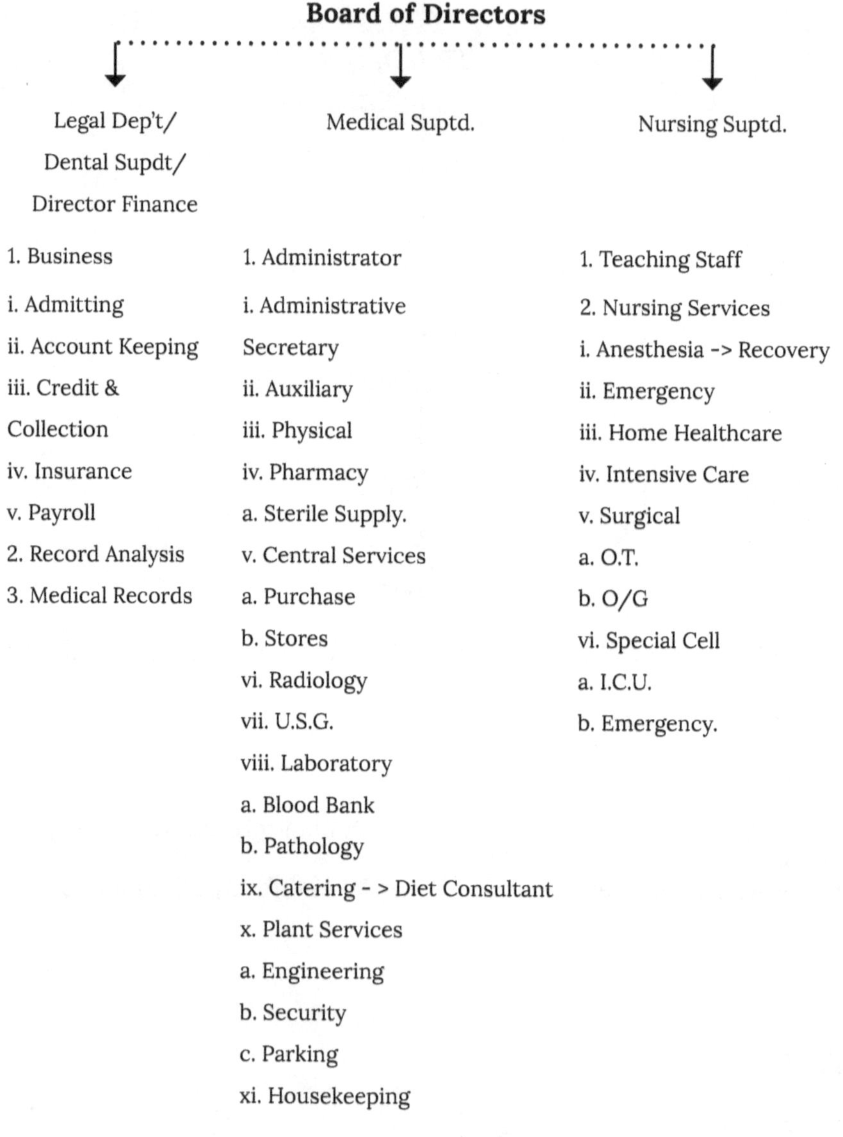

Many service departments have been working since long, but to come up to the mark they have to work harder and still harder.

3) ***Infrastructure development:***

Infrastructure development is also one of the priority areas which requires an action plan & development of specific work culture. Specific requirements are there both at-

   a)   Composite Hospital level.&

   b)   Bn., SHQ. FTR. HQ, FHQ Medical Inspection Rooms & Hospitals if any(52).

A time bound action plan is a must which should be adhered to especially for the development of infrastructure at different levels .As such infrastructure, man & material development go hand in hand in restructuring of Medical Set up in CPMFs as well as SSB. Constraints are there but development has to take place in spite of all odds. Development of infrastructure as such of composite hospital level is called for and a detailed discussion is called for in this regard, which is a big topic for discussion in itself.

4)   **Economics involvement-Freshinitiatives.**

A fresh initiative is required to complete the pending infrastructure requirements and newer initiative

(54) for infrastructure development, for Pathology, for Pharmacy and Hospital equipments purchase and maintenance.

Though funds are being pumped on a regular interval but it requires a solid base to have our own setup which cannot be developed without the finances being at our beck and call.

2.2.3 Third phase (2008 – 2010 & further) Theme: Deployment of SSB on IBB

Sashastra Seema Bal (SSB) placed under the **Ministry of Home Affairs, Government of India as a Central Para Military Force (CPMF)** was also deployed on the **Indo Bhutan Border (IBB) in the year 2008.**

Chapter 3
REVIEW OF LITERATURE

3.1 INTRODUCTION:

Strategic planning positions an organization for long-term sustainability and high stakeholder value. Strategic planners ask questions such as what business are we in? What is our corporate culture? And where are changes taking place in the market? The well-thought out strategic plan also provides answers to many of those questions with vision and mission statements, goals, objectives, and action plans.

The strategic plan is the overall guide to the development and growth of the organization. A strategic plan is a long-range plan, usually done every three to ten years. Strategic plans can be prepared on many levels of the organization as well. There may be functional plans, site plans, business unit plans, and so on. Each lower-level plan rolls up until it is incorporated into the top-most organization plan. Annual operating plans are built to support the strategic plan. These annual plans deal with monetary and staffing requirements.

In order to decide where the company is going and how it will get there, top management, Kerzner (2001)said:

1. It scans the external environment and industrial environment for changing conditions.

2. Interprets the changing environment in terms of opportunities or threats.

3. Analyzes the firm's resource base for assessing strengths and weaknesses.

4. Defines the mission of the business by matching environmental opportunities and threats with resource strengths and weaknesses.

Sets goals for pursuing the mission based on top management values and sense of responsibility. (p. 15)

During the study for developing a strategic plan for effective health services for SSB the following Methodology was followed –

1) Direct– (a) Survey of personnel from Sashastra SeemaBal.

      (b) Survey of beneficiaries outside the ambit of Sashastra Seema Bal.

2) Indirect (Published works) –

      a) Books (Literature survey).

      b) Research reports - review there of.

      c) Survey reports.

      d) Committee reports.

      e) Journal reports.

      f) Analysis of policy documents.

In this chapter a review of published work in the form of Literature Survey, Research reports, Survey reports, committee reports and journal reports has been studied to form a base for Effective Health services for SSB.

SSB on the borders is involved in multitasking like cordon and search operations, apprehending drug traffickers, hot pursuit of smugglers day in and day out. Occasionally this involves round the clock even at night manning the borders leading to ill health of the jawans and their families.

3.2 (a) Books (Literature survey):

As such in order to reach an effective strategic plan for SSB health services during the conceptualization phase what exactly were the views of the learned and well established authors was looked into. **A literature survey was carried out specially related with the review of the following books (Indirect Method)–**

1. Strategic planning for public and non profit organization.

2. An international assessment of health care –Financial Aspects.

3. Health services research - Ananthology.

4. Health care in Asia.

5. India – Economic development and Social opportunity.

   Further in this indirect survey of literature the following reports were also taken into account –

a) Research reports – review thereof (case study- eg- Getwell Hospital, IGIMS, CMCH Vellore and PMCH Patna,NBMCH-RDA-Slg)

b) Survey reports.

c) Committee reports.

d) Journal reports.

e) Analysis of policy documents.

3.2 (a) (1)   Strategic planning for public and non profit organization:

Strategic planning for public and non profit organization is a book written by **John M. Bryson** who suggest that Strategic planning indicators for a Government or not for profit Organization are more in number and perhaps more ambiguous than those of private for profit organization.

The book studies in depth strategic planning for –

a)   Future direction.

b)   Priorities action to betaken.

c)   Formulating guidelines to apply the process.

d)   The need of studying strategic planning.

e)   Developing coherent and defendable basis for decision making.

f)   Exercising discretion in areas under organizational control.

Overall the book provides a basic guideline in strategic planning for an organization through which SSB Health Services can benefit.

3.2 (a) (2)   An international assessment of health care – Financial Aspects:

DAVID W. DUNLOP and JO. M. MARTINS [ED-SEMINAR SERIES] in their book *"An International Assessment of Health Care – Financial Aspects"* have the following to advice policy makers in developing countries–

Welfare of the society – View of the society.

Public and Private arrangements for financing schemes. Effective resource allocation.

In a few societies to protect the benefits for the patient a licensing system for medical practitioners is provided to ensure minimum standards at the entry level. However this can result into a single (Monopoly) or a few (Oligopoly) producers who have the power to influence the price and quantity of service provided.

CONCLUSIONS:

Health financing -- evolutionary in nature.

The characteristics of the health care market on both the supply and demand side suggest the presence of market failure conditions or vice versa.

Health financing policy has three ultimate concerns- Equity and efficiency.

Free price setting and consumer choice. Budgetary constraints.

Health financing can be done through a variety of mechanisms like :

Tax Financing.

Premiums for Health Scheme users.

Private-public mix of ownership in health care delivery.

Establishment of mechanisms and facilities to gather relevant information in an efficient manner are necessary in implementing the health financing policy.

Rationing of health services in the absence of unlimited resources or due to budgetary constraints. Finally, more work can and should be done to enrich the available resources to the policy makers.

3.2 (a) (3)   Health services research - Ananthology:

3.1.3(a)   Medical auditing by scientific methods illustrated by major female pelvic surgery.

- PAUL A. LEMBEKE, M.D.

To have a strategic plan, finances too have a role to play.

"...... the purpose of medical auditing is to make certain that the full benefits of medical knowledge are being applied effectively to the needs of the patients." (Pg. 99)

"...... health care which reduces mortality, however also raises the output of workers in a nation by increasing the vitality of these workers, many diseases with high prevalence rates in underdeveloped nations like malaria etc are chief cripplers of mankind rather than killers.

"...... A strategy should be formulated to kill these organisms in the health care scenario everytime when it comes to developing such a strategy." (Pg. 254)

3.2.3(b)   Medical care : Its social and organizational aspects. Health service systems in the US and other countries critical comparisons.

ODIN W. ANDERSON PH.D.

" in all countries, the hospital and the clinics attached for outpatient services became the main site for the care of the low income patients and the indigent. Physicians normally provided their services free because the hospital was the only place where the latest medical techniques and knowledge were being introduced systematically, it was a place where such techniques and knowledge could be applied to relatively large number of patients."

"... it is clothed with public interest." (Pg. 261)

"... health insurance is evolving in a certain direction." (Pg. 263)

In the USA

"... 70% population covered by certain type of insurance."

"... govt. on various levels provides care for special groups such as veterans, MCH and special diseases such as mental illness and tuberculosis."

"...federalgovernmenthasassistedsince1946ingrantstothestatesf o r the construction, expansion and renovation of general hospitals, but not in payment for services." (Pg.264)

In Sweden

"... Enrolment in government sponsored health insurance is mandatory for total population."

"... health service system is financed from a variety of services."

> Payments from employers and employees.

> Direct charges to patients

> Funds from country and municipal governments for general hospital care.

> Funds from the federal government for mental and tuberculosis hospitals.

As such it can be expected that approximately 65% of the funds come from governmental sources. (Pg. 264)

In U.K.

"...nearly the whole population has virtually free access to private health services just by signing up with a general practitioner. 95% have already signed."

"All services and goods are provided by the system, and almost the whole of the health system is owned and operated by the central government."

<u>Special emphasis is on:</u>

> Entire cost paid from general tax funds collected by the CGHS. (Only a small portion is paid by pay roll deductions.)

> Patients must be refereed by general physicians, who don't have hospital appointments, unlike specialists who are salaried members of the medical staff.

> Prescription drugs are provided at a small charge for prescriptions and pharmacists are paid according to a schedule arrived at by negotiation with the government.

(Pg.264-65)

3.2.3*(c)*   *Epidemiology of Family Practice:*

- R.R. HUNTLEY, M.D.

"... Primary, personal, medical care is not given entirely by general practitioners. The NDTI (National Disease and Therapeutic Index) reports that American internists see only 23% of their patients on referral from other physicians."

" ... This study can be utilized to delineate the area of responsibility of the family's personnel physician, thereby indicating the body of knowledge which must be transmitted to those preparing to enter this field." (Pg.269)

(While formulating a strategic plan for health care workers and systems such research and study should be incorporated).

3.2.3(d)   *Case Fatality in Teaching and Non – Teaching Hospitals:*

- L. LIPWORTH; J.A.H. LEE; J.N. MORRIS

"... Difference in case fatality represents superior treatment in the teaching hospitals."

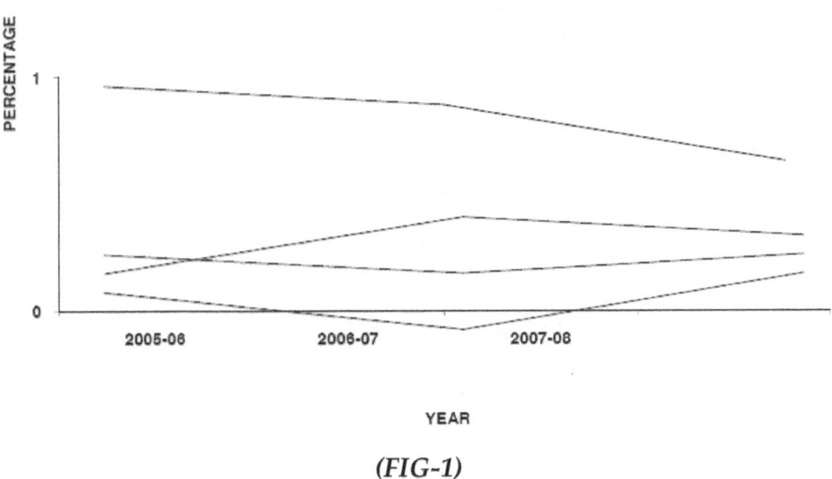

(FIG-1)

LineNo.1 : Teaching (Appendicitis with Peritonitis)

LineNo.2 : Teaching (Hyperplasia ofProstate)

LineNo.3 : Non Teaching (Appendicitis with Peritonitis)

LineNo.4 : Non Teaching (Hyperplasia of Prostate)

Case fatality of Hyperplasia of Prostate, Appendicitis with Peritonitis in Teaching & Non Teaching Hospitals

A strategy can be developed to augment the existing hospital facilities for in-house, on the job training and practice sessions especially in the case of a strategy to be followed at the Frontier and Functional level of SSBHS.

" ... The non-teaching hospital patients may be socially or otherwise be at an initial disadvantage. It has already been shown that proportionate to their number of beds, teaching hospitals had more consultants and other staff." (Pg. 231).

Hospital staffing should be reviewed accordingly while augmenting the strategic plan for SSB health services.

3.2.3(e) *Decision Rules, Types of Error, and their Consequences in Medical Diagnosis :*

- THOMAS J. SCHEFF

"... Diagnosis and treatment are influenced by the pay off for the clinician (Read Psychiatrist) as well as for the patient." (Pg. 304)

As such a mutually beneficial strategic plan should be formulated in any health care organization be it SSB or its external environment players since care through doctors is bound to be there.

3.2.3(f) *The Hazards of Hospitalization:*

"... A judicious selection of diagnostic and therapeutic measures can be made only with the knowledge of potential hazards as well as the proposed benefits." (Pg.322)

The strategy formulation involving the concerned physicians should be provided in view of the above mentioned hazards of hospitalization.

3.2.3(g) *Stages of Illness and Medical Care:*

- E.A. SUCHMAN

To have an idea of "Stages of Illness and Medical Care" and their effect on strategy planning the five stages representing major transition points are:

1. The symptom experience stage.

2. The assumption of the sick role stage.

3. The medical care contact stage.

4. The dependent patient role stage.

5. The recovery of rehabilitation stage.

After going into the intricacies of all these five stages it was found that we don't know about those cases in the community which may require them. However, those receiving it are adequately treated". (Pg. 336-37).**In the strategic planning process one should as such concentrate on the most vulnerable in the society getting adequate medical coverage. (Remote areas of INB & IBB can be covered by SSB under this strategy).**

3.2.3(h) *Why People use Health Services:*

- I.M. ROSENSTOCK

" ... Since health decisions are determined by a variety of personal, interpersonal and situational factors, attempts to induce people to change their health actions may successfully be undertaken at various points in the decision process." (Pg. 380)**Minimizing barriers to action, maximizing convenience and providing intensive cues to action are suggested for incorporation in the strategic plan for SSB Health Services.**

3.2.3(i) *The Medical Audit as an Operational Tool:*

- M.A. MOREHEAD M.D.

"... Cases were selected at random from the admitting office of the OPD. ... A major weakness was   shown to exist by the lack of co-ordination between specialty departments. For example, a woman was followed for more than six year by the ophthalmology department where she went frequently for new glasses. Fundus examination reports over the years showed increasing evidence of degenerative changes and vascular disease. However, it was not until the sixth years when the women suffered a stroke that she came to the attention of the department." (Pg.392)

By similar shifts in case selection this method of physician appraisal of clinical handling of medical records can be used to meet different objectives. **The regular CME classes will help in such cases.**

The content of the reviews can be compiled to examine both administrative and professional strategies.

3.2.3(j)   *Activities, Events and Outcomes in Ambulatory Patient Care:*

- C.E. LEWIS M.D. : D. WAXMAN M.D.

"... Although there were no differences in terms of deaths or severity of disease between the two patient groups (nurse clinics and control groups) there were statistically significant difference in outcomes in terms of reduction of disability and relative decrease in discomfort and dissatisfaction of patients seen in the ambulatory clinic. (Pg.444).

The ambulatory care service should be incorporated in the strategic plan when formed.

3.2.3(k)   *Health Services Research – A Working Model*

- B. STORFIELD, M.D.

" ... The field of health services is concerned with the application of biomedical knowledge to prevent, treat, control and eliminate disease and to restore function and minimize disability.

3.2.3(l)   *The Marriage of Primary Care and Epidemiology:*

"... There is no practical way for literally millions of patients to benefit from application of the highest standards except through use of structured information to acquire an adequate communication technique to transmit rapidly the appropriate information." (Pg.561).

3.2.3*(m)* ***The Organization of Medical Practice and Practice Orientations among Physicians in Prepaid and Non-prepaid Primary Care Settings***

- DAVID MECHANIC PH.D.

"... The problem is inherent in the fact that the number of physician hours available relative to patient demand is low in capitation and prepaid practice." (Pg.614).

Strategy planning can take care of increasing physician hours.

3.2.4 Health care in Asia:

Health care in Asia is a fast and furiously growing enterprise which is taking a shape of a multimillion dollar business. As per Global Health situations and projections of WHO (3) different research oriented programs are an ongoing process which suggest the following-

i   Performance varies from country to country. Variability is large at places.

ii   Improved policy decisions can help increase female life expectancy, especially in countries like India, China, Myanmar & Sri Lanka. (ReferExhibit-1).

iii   Females live longer in all countries of the world except in India, Nepal &Bangladesh.

iv   Targeting infectious and parasitic diseases amongst children in developing countries would also help reduce death rates in all other age groups.

v   Private expenditure on health care plays an important role in all countries but in India, Indonesia, Korea, Myanmar, the Philippines and Thailand private spending accounts for more than half the total.

vi   India's relatively high spending on health much of which is out of pocket spending by individuals & state governments, raises some policy issues unique to its situation.

Two of the most important health issues are the-

a)   Women up to the age of 45 have poor health outcomes.

b)   Infant Mortality Rate is high in some areas of the country.

Are central government funds channeled into these areas? Are public health activities the first priority for these funds? The evidence suggests that the allocation of central government funds does not target these persistent problems. Maternal and child health services receive only 20 percent of the amount the central government spends to train physicians (4, 5).

(Table 1-A, B, C, D show the pattern of spending on programs and distribution of central government allocation for Health Services in India.)

Research Priorities:

1.   Population Programmes to be analyzed similarly.

2.   Factors like health care, price of drugs and medical supplies, capital required and cost of training personnel require further research.

3.   Lack of Knowledge regarding output from budgets for public health activities and curative health activities.

Exhibit – 1

Female and Male Life Expectancy and Infant Mortality Rates (IIMR)

Female Life Expectancy	Female	Male	IMR per 1000
Nepal	47	48	130
Bangladesh	50	51	121
India	56	57	86
Indonesia	58	55	87

TABLE 1-A

State Characteristic and Health and Family Welfare Expenditure in India.

(Around Late 80's and Early 90's)

Sl. No.	State	Per Capita Income (Rs.) 1983-84)	Plan Per Capita Expenditure (Rs.)	Non-plan Per Capita Expenditure (Rs.)	Total Per Capita Expenditure (Rs.)
1.	Assam	1,762	6	11	17
2.	Bihar	1,174	5	08	13
3.	Haryana	3,147	11	14	24
4.	H.P.	2,230	29	31	60
5.	J &K.	1,820	09	32	41

Note: (i)   It is a sample of States.

          (ii) Those with incomplete data have been left out.

Source: (i)   Income and population - Kristen 1988, Tables 1 &2.

          (ii) Expenditure - Rao, Kahn and Prasad 1987.

States with higher incomes tend to spend more on health and family welfare. However, the relationship between income and spending is not strong. But the total range in spending is large. Himanchal Pradesh, with per capita income of 2,230 rupees spends the most, nearly five times more per person than Bihar, with per capita income of 1,174 rupees. Trends for J&K are similar in nature.

TABLE 1-B

Distribution of State spending o onn Health Care, India (In %)

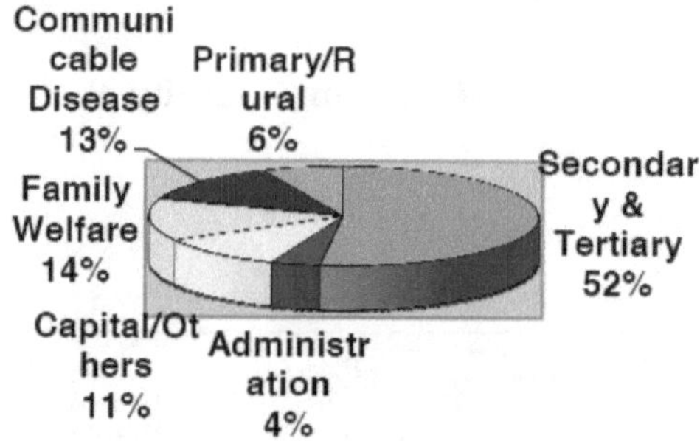

It is important to state that the most expensive hospitals and training facilities be put in urban areas if they are to be utilized properly and employ specialized labor. In the more densely populated countries of Asia, locating these facilities in urban areas is less important than it is in the more populated countries of Africa and Latin America, but nowhere are hospitals put in wilderness (5, 6). Thus, hospital spending in an urban setup is quite inevitable and generally reflects economic necessity more than spending less on a district setup.

TABLE 1-C

HEALTH SERVICES EXPENSES BY PROGRAMME IN INDIA

Sl. No.	Program	State Spending	Govt. Spending	Total
1.	Administrative	4.0	1.6	3.7
2.	Sec. & Tertiary	39.3	6.1	34.7
	Medical Relief			
	Insurance	6.4	8.7	6.7
	Medical Education	6.1	15.2	7.4
3.	Primary/Rural			
	Paramedical Training	1.2	1.4	1.2
	Rural Health	4.5	0.7	4
	MCH	1.0	2.9	1.3
4.	Communicable Disease	12.8	4.5	11.6
5.	School Health	0.1	0	0.1
6.	Family Planning	13.8	20.7	14.8
7.	Other	8.1	11.2	8.5
8.	Capital	2.7	26.9	6.1
9.	Total	100	99.9	100
10.	Rupees(Thousands)	14,763,400	2,388,535	17,151,935
11.	Percentage of Total	86	14	100

64% of expenditure will be consumed by hospitals when family planning is removed and administration and capital allocated to each programme.

Similarly, expenditure increases annually as per the chart prepared above depending on the plan outlay.

TABLE 1-D

DISTRIBUTION OF CENTRAL GOVT. ALLOCATION FOR HEALTH SERVICES IN INDIA (IN %)

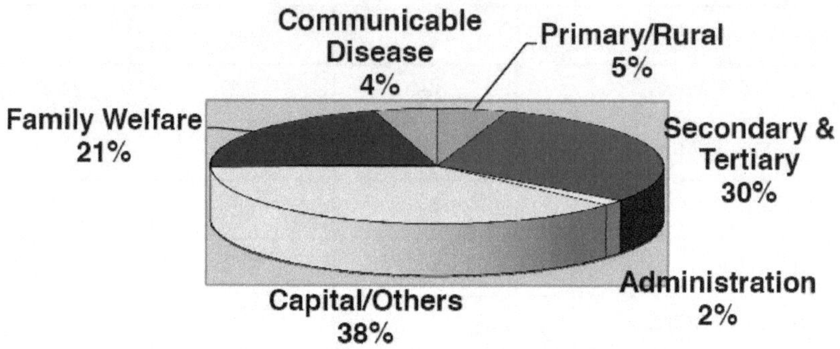

Distribution of Health Care Expenditure between Urban and Rural Areas in India

Sl. No.	State	Urban	Rural	Common	Urban Bias
1.	Assam	33.6	21.2	45.2	3.7
2.	Bihar	23.5	28.4	48.1	2.4
3.	Haryana	43.3	19.5	37.2	2.4
4.	H.P.	22.0	25.6	52.4	3.4
5.	J & K	52.5	18.1	29.4	2.8

Urban bias in spending is seen via these charts. Spending is more and pronounced compared to the rural entity in the urban areas which most probably is profit based and market orient d. considerable discretion is exercised as to where and how funds are to be spent –in this case urban area. The state too is encouraged for urban spending. The biases can be correlated through a number of policy decisions like-Ceiling on urban spending should be there. Rural upliftment should be the key in the future policy decisions. Insurance and user fees from urban areas be utilized in rural area disease control. Individual should benefit only after the community & Expenses are retargeted.

3.2 (a) (5)   India – Economic development and Social opportunity

The development of the country depends on the social opportunity provided by a host of activities interlinked with action originating from economics (5). India is no exception to the rule.

A few important aspects related with it are as follows-

i   "... Economic reforms are a must in the present scenario". (Pg.202).

ii   "... The expansion of markets is among the instruments that can help to promote human capabilities and given the imperative need for rapid elimination of endemic deprivation in India, it would be irresponsible to ignore that opportunity." (Pg.203).

iii   "... There is a strong case for taking adequate note of the tremendous social and economic deprivations that blight living conditions in India and limit the actual prospects of participatory economic expansion." (Pg.204).

Strategies and policies should be formulated in such a way that the above pointers may be incorporated for further development and upliftment of the common man at large. SSB has worked with aplomb in the state of J&K very recently and the experience of working there has helped them on the INB as well. A few features related with J&K can be simulated for mutual benefit on the INB which are as follows:

1.	Population	1991	8 millions (Projected from earlier year).
2.	Death Rate	1990-92	8.0 (1988-90) (For three year average).
3.	Birth Rate	1990-92	31.5 (For three year average).
4.	Total Fertility Rate	1991	3.3 (For three year average).
5.	Literacy and Edu. (%)	1992-93	F-37.7; M-56.3 (Jammu only).
6.	School attendance and enrolment (%)	1986-87	Rural : F-47.6;M-21.5
			Urban : F-29.3; M- 18.9
7.	Female employment(%)	1989	9.5 (In Public Sector)
8.	Proportion of Villages with medical facilities	1981	17.9 (%)
9.	Proportion of households having access to safe drinking water (%)	1991	Rural-60.9; Urban-82.8
10.	No. of hospital beds per million persons	1991	Rural-77 ; Urban-4,215.

iv   Ratio of female to male child mortality among Hindus and Muslims in different States,Emphasis – J & K- 1981 (Extrapolation for 1991).

3.2(b) Research reports - review thereof:

1.   A research report related with **Strategic Changes in Hospitals- an examination** *provided the following findings-*

    a)   Hospitals sampled-

        i.   Investor owned.

        ii.   Not for profit hospitals.

        iii.   Free standing hospitals.

        iv.   Members of multi hospital systems.

        v.   Hospitals of all sizes.

    b)   Strategic change evaluated by classifying strategy type in-

        i.   Each of the two consecutive five year time periods (1980-85 and1986-90).

        ii.   Change in reimbursement policies.

        iii.   Emergence of new technologies.

        iv.   Changing customer expectations.

        v.   New sources of competition.

All these made the environment for hospitals progressively more turbulent in the latter period and provided an opportune setting to evaluate strategic change.

Results suggested that a significant number of hospitals did change strategy as the environment changed and in the direction anticipated.

Logistic regression was used to determine whether –

> ➢ Prior Strategy
>
> ➢ Type of ownership
>
> ➢ System membership or
>
> ➢ Size

Would predict which hospitals would change strategy as the environment changed. "Only prior strategy was found to be a predictor of strategy change." .... **Strategic Change in hospitals: An examination of the response of the acute care hospital to the turbulent environment of the 1980's.- HEALTH SERVICE RESEARCH 1990 – OCT 25(4):565-91**

2.   "Hospitals face a set of issues critical to strategy formulation that are markedly different than those faced by traditional corporations, divisions or functional areas. Given this, the relevance of current business approaches to strategy formulation that focus exclusively on a narrowest of market driven factors is questionable."

"Hospitals, it is argued must take a more comprehensive view of strategy formulation that goes beyond issues of internal competency and environmental opportunities to incorporate the values of care givers and the societal responsibilities of the institution as well". **...Formulating Hospital Strategy: Moving beyond a market mentality. Rutgers University, New Brunswick, N. J.**

- (HEALTH CARE MANAGEMENT REVIEW 1992-WINTER; 17(1):21-6)

3.   ***Uncompensated hospital care – Will it be there if we need it?***

DEPARTMENT OF HEALTH CARE POLICY HARVARD MEDICAL SCHOOL, BOSTON-USA.

"The debate over health care system reform continue, but they rarely mention the enduring need for free or reduced cost hospital care as a safety net for uninsured and underinsured individuals." The changes on multiple fronts threaten the ability or willingness of hospitals to provide for uncompensated care.

This may lead to decline of funds, closing or merger of not for profit & public hospitals, competitive forces dominating the market and so on.

"Measurement of uncompensated care is inconsistent "... policies need to be re-examined".

"... guidelines for policy based on past experience are presented herein".

...**WEISSMAN J. (JAMA –1996 SEPT–11; 276 (10): 823-8)**

4.   ***Economic regulation and hospital behavior: The effects of medical staff organization and hospital physician relationships–***

    i   New forms of payment.

    ii   Growing competition.

    iii   Controlled evolution of multi-unit hospital systems.

    iv   Associated forces.

are redefining the fundamental relationship between hospitals and physicians. Results arrived at by examining –

    i   Cross-sectional data.

    ii   Data collected at two points in time.

Regulation and competition- findings suggest - at least upto 1982- had relatively little direct effect on hospital medical staff and organization.

Changes are more strongly associated with –

    i   Hospital care mix.

    ii   Structural characteristics involving membership in a multi unit system, size, ownership and location.

"The persuasive effect of case mix and the consistent effect of multi unit system involvement support the need for policy makers to give these factors particular attention in considering how hospitals and their medical staffs might respond to future –

    ➤ Regulatory, &or

    ➤ Competitive approaches

-SHORTEIISM; MORRISEYMA; CONCRADDA (HEALTH SERVICERES–1985-DEC; 20(5); 597-628)

5. ***Do not resuscitate policies in Midwestern hospitals: A five state survey–***

    i   States-   Five Midwestern States.

    ii   Institutions   -986.

    iii   Respondents Percentage -76.

    iv   Results–

        a.   DNR -35.5%.

        b.   In the process of developing DNR policies -24.4%.

        c.   Ethical committees -38.1%.

v   Variables associated with the results-

        a.   Institutional size.

        b.   Existence of an ethics committee.

vi   Recommendations-

        a.   Further Research required.

b)   Study of ethical problems in medicine and biomedical and behavioral research.

- MOZDZIER GJ; SCHLESINGER SE (HEALTH SERV RES 1986, FET, 20 (6 PT 2): 949-60)

4.   ***The effects of corporate re-structuring on hospital policy making–***

"Hospital corporate re-structuring is the segmentation of assets or functions of the hospital into separate corporations or divisions."

The Study Examines:

i   Effect of corporate re-structuring by community hospitals on the

      – Structure

      – Composition

      – Activity of hospital governing boards.

      – Policy making function of the hospital will change to adapt to the multi corporate/ divisional strategy implemented under corporate re-structuring.

Analysis done by –

ii   Survey data from 1,037 hospitals undergoing corporate re-structuring from1979-85.

iii A comparison group of 1,883 none corporately re-structured hospitals suggesting general support for this hypothesis.

N.B.: This has been finally incorporated as the Strategic plan for SSB Health Services with special reference to INB. However,a mix between the two is definitely on the agenda.

- ALEXANDER JA; MORLOCK LL; GIFFORD BD, (DEPARTMENT OF HEALTH SERVICE ADMINISTRATION, UNIVERSITY OF ALABAMA, BIRMINGHAN)

5. ***Legal issues in determining competence to make treatment decisions***.

- BENESCH K

" ... Psychiatrists are increasingly called on to evaluate patients' competence to make treatment decisions".

- NEW DIR. MENT. HEALTH SERV-1989 – SPRING; (41):97–105.

6. ***Hospital policy on advance directives. Do institutions ask patients about living wills?***

➢ Survey suggests substantial proportion of the population has proposed for advance directive.

➢ To assess existence and nature of hospital policy regarding these documents.

➢ Survey Questionnaire; 394 randomly selected hospitals in USA.

➢ Response from219.

➤ Policy.

i. Formal policy 146(67%) (For Advance Directive)

ii. Patients Enquiry 4% (Actively)

iii. Ethical committee 46% of the respondents.

- Ethical/ legal issues regarding hospital policy on advance directives are discussed.

Hospitals should adopt formal policies to ask all adult patients at the time of admission whether they have prepared a living will, durable power of attorney, or similar document and ethical committee should play a more active role in policy development.

DEPARTMENT OF HEALTH POLICY AND MANAGEMENT, JOHNS HOPKINS UNIVERSITY SCHOOL OF HYGIENE AND PUBLIC HEALTH, BALTIMORE. MCCRARY SV: BOTKINJR.

7. ***Nursing Administration and personnel Administration–***

"... Numerous nursing directors and hospital administrators expressed a desire for more support for the personnel department, but their priorities concerning the degree of increased involvement differed".

"... Managers at all levels will find this article to be a fruitful basis for discussing those areas within which the personnel department could play an expanded role".

- WHITE HC; WOLFE MN; (J NURS ADM 1983 JUL-AUG.; 13 (7-8):15-9

3.2(c) Survey Reports:

1. A student from Kent, K.Dasmis speaks of a strategic plan which is a must for any health service organization because of the following drawbacks:

    i. Appointments being badly scheduled.

    ii. OPD clinics create a large pool of patients in the initial stage.

    iii. Emergency plan required for patients arriving in the emergency.

2. A UK survey concludes that–

    i. Co-ordination must between the OPD & teaching students.

    ii. Clinicians, consultants and patients have insufficient space.

    iii. Alternative arrangements when medical staff is on leave is insufficient.

    iv. Clinics poorly organized.

    v. Distribution of labor-uneven.

    vi. Patient referrals –unwarranted-mostly by General Physicians.

In the context of SSBHS it is further noted that the points as illustrated in the UK survey are to be addressed properly whether it is patient referral or OPD management or distribution of labour or alternative arrangements when the medical staff is on leave.

3.2(d) Committee Reports:

1. *National Institute of Health and Family Welfare (NIHFW),* New Delhi) suggests a few remedial features (1995-96) which are as follows:

    a. Hospital buildings and its different wings be planned properly.

    b. Patients to be screened for admission.

    c. Tick what is wanted in the Printed Investigation form to save precious time.

    d. Drugs to be packed to save time at the pharmacy counter.

    e. Appointment system.

2. *Jain Committee (1968)*

    Suggestions include:

    a. A strategic plan to see old and new cases.

        New cases -Morning

        Old cases - Evening

    b. Satellite OPDs required.

    c. Junior doctors to screen patients.

    d. Establish polyclinics in the adjacent areas of big hospitals.

    e. Family doctors to have diagnostic facilities.

3. *International Consultation, CMC, Vellore*

    The Director, B.M. Pulimood points (7) to challenges to be faced by the institution in the 1990's as:

    i.   Health care to have a holistic approach.

    ii. Services at Primary, Secondary and Tertiary levels of referral in health care should be properly integrated.

    iii. Maintaining financial autonomy for cost effective service.

    iv. Research should be need based.

    The purpose is to give healing and wholeness, rather than simply a cure for which an extensive system of communication may have to be developed on an emergency basis.

4. *Timmappaya (1968):*

    A proper signposting of different departments is suggested..

5. *Recommendations of Management Science Staff of University of kent-*

    f. Start OPD on time.

    a. Pool fewer patients.

    b. Patients to be better scheduled.

    c. Waiting area should be proper.

    d. Hospitals to have –

        (i) Proper diagnostic facilities;

        (ii) Proper Medical records facility.

3.2(e) Journal Reports:

1.   *Leading an ear to the customer:*

"Successful companies have oriented themselves towards customers, responding to their tastes and ordering their strategies towards their total satisfaction".

- MARKET ORIENTATION; HUND AND MORGAN –1995

According to them –

i   The systematic gathering of information on customers and competitors, both present and potential.

ii   The analysis of such information for building up knowledge for the profit of the customer.

iii   Strategy formulation and implementation by use of such knowledge.

"*Janki Raman* (1995) further signed market (Read Health Care) orientation based on the level of contest the organization can exercise. Consumer (patients) has been segregated as internal and external consumers."

"Capabilities are complex bundles of skills and collective learning exercised through the organizational process that ensure superior co-ordination of functional activities."

"Market orientation "can be restated as –

i   Information Generation from all customers viz

- Internal and External

- Present and Future

ii   Inter- functional co-ordination.

iii   Consumers requirements to be responded to.

    iv   Informed consent to the consumers.

    v   Generate continuous information for consumers.

Crystallization has-however not yet been achieved.

"Payne (1988) suggests a programme based on successful case studies increasing market orientation."

    i   Potentially conflicting orientations should be understood

    ii   Evaluating the present levels of market effectiveness.

    iii   For the improvement of the market, implementation of different plans be made.

However, according to Slater and Narver (1994) –

"The rebuttable presumption is that business (Real Health Organization (Strategic Plan) that is more market oriented is best positioned for success under any environmental conditions. Being market oriented is the basis for creating superior value for buyers, the meaning of competitive advantage. Accordingly, a strategy having market orientation can never negate.

M. JANAKIRAMAN (PROF-IIM-LUCKNOW) (IN INDIAN
MANAGEMENT AUGUST -1997; 30-34)

2.   *Public hospitals under contract management – An assessment of operating performance*

"Private organizations are managing mostly because of serious fiscal deterioration".

The study examines the effects of these contract management arrangements on the operating performance of public hospitals which pales into insignificance compared to private players.

Performance areas considered are --

    i   Efficiency of operation.

    ii   Service structure.

    iii   Medicare/medic-aid caseload

JEFFREY A. ALEXANDER, PH. D; THOMAS G. RUNDALL, PH.D
(MEDICAL CARE 1985, 23;209-19)

3.   *Health Service Research and Quality of Care:*

For the 1990s the basics should include –

Health care managers, purchasers and regulators.

Health services research must pursue at least three intellectual agenda which are as follows:

    i   The study of efficacy (Knowing what works)

    ii   The study of appropriateness (Using what works)

    iii   The study of the execution of care (Doing well what works).

The responsibility for the financing and conduct of the research agendas varies with the level of segregation of data and effort needed for each topic.

The three topics must be pursued effectively if health care quality is to be successfully defined, measured and protected.

DONALD M. BERWICK, M.D. (MED. CARE – 1989; 27:763-771)

3.2(f) Analysis of policy documents

3.2(f)(i) INTRODUCTION:

Effective health services for the nation are not only the prerogative of the Central Government but the nation at large.

Not only the Central Government, but the different departments under it are also involved to shoulder the responsibility among themselves. SSB, ITBP, CRPF, BSF & the Army are a few examples who are involved in this specific work.

The Area of responsibility is their field of work related with health care. SSB, as such is involved in and around Indo Nepal Border where it provides medical cover to the needy villagers on a need basis. Malaria is quite prevalent on the foothills of Darjeeling District where SSB is of prime importance. It is   for their own benefit and for the benefit of the society at large that these policy decisions-directly or indirectly- are involved with the health services of all CPMFs. SSB- as such, has a leading role to play in the control of these health hazards.

During the phase wise development of the building blocks for effective health service for SSB- analysis of policy documents was also carried out to develop a specific plan for the final out come to be   incorporated for Sashastra Seema Bal. Some of the policy documents that were analyzed are as follows : **3.2(f)(ii) Analysis of policy documents:**

3.2 (f)(ii)(1) NATIONAL MALARIA ERADICATION/ CONTROL PROGRAMME:

The National Concern: NMCP or "National Malaria Control Programme" was launched in 1953 to reduce the incidence of Malaria in India.

From more than 75 million cases in 1952 it was brought down to 2 million cases in 1958.

However, NMCP was up graded to NMEP, i.e. "National Malaria Eradication Programme" since it was envisioned that insect vectors might develop resistance to insecticides. NMEP was started in 1958.

An all time low was achieved in 1961, amounting to about 50,000 cases only. However the above figures could not be sustained because of -

   i   Administrative

   ii   Operational

   iii   Technical

   iv   Social

   v   Economic&

   vi   Human factors million cases with 59 deaths.

relegating the figures into doldrums. This includes 6.4

Later, a modified plan of operations, NMCP was put into action with effect from 1st April, 1977. Incidence of malaria (8) declined there after each year. Against 6.4 million cases in 1971 only 1.7 million cases were recorded in 1986. As such a reduction of about 70% was seen.

However, a gradual augmentation (9) of P. falciparum was seen during this time, as such a programme to limit P. falciparum was also launched during this time.

The commitment of "Health for All" by the Government of India has led to inclusion/integration of (10) "Anti Malaria Activity" with "Primary Health Care."(PHC).

PHC committees are involved in collection & examination of blood smears from fever cases through multipurpose workers. Community participation in remote and rural areas is a must and emphasized too.

The drug distribution centers are manned by –

    i   Panchayat Members

    ii   Forest officials

    iii   Village health guides&

    iv   Other community workers

The Fever treatment depots are manned by–

    i   Traders

    ii   Forest

    iii   Revenue officials.

Insecticide spraying operations are supervised by "District Malaria officials".

Here the work of SSB health service comes into play especially-

    a)   Collection & examination of Blood smears

    b)   Drug distribution

    c)   Fever treatment

    d)   Insecticide spraying operation-

Which all can be coordinated by the help of SSB hospital Para Medical Staff and Doctors, Lab/Tech and Pharmacists.

MALARIA ACTION PLAN (MAP):

An expert committee on Malaria came into being in 1994 with the following objectives-

    a)   Complicated case management of Malaria.

    b)   High Risk group vulnerable to mortality- prevention there of.

c)   Epidemic and out break control.

d)   Control of drug resistant malaria.

e)   P. falciparum incidence reduction.

f)   Low incidence status maintenance.

MALARIA WEEK:

Occasional resurgence of malaria in different parts of the country has regenerated the need for strengthening health promotion for all. As such from "1st of May to 7th of May" every year "Malaria Week "is observed.

The main aim is to create awareness among the masses about malaria and its prevention. The SSB Scenario:

Action plan required especially in the foothills of Sikkim, Darjeeling in West Bengal, Bihar, U.P, UttaraKhand on IndoNepal Border and on Indo Bhutan Border – Assam foothills which are quite prone to mosquito menace and therefore malaria.

3.2 (f)(ii) (2) NATIONAL FILARIA CONTROL PROGRAMME (NFCP):

According to a National Survey of 1955.

a)   People at Risk – 420million.

b)   People Manifesting disease – 19million.

c)   People having parasite in Blood – 25million.

Two components of

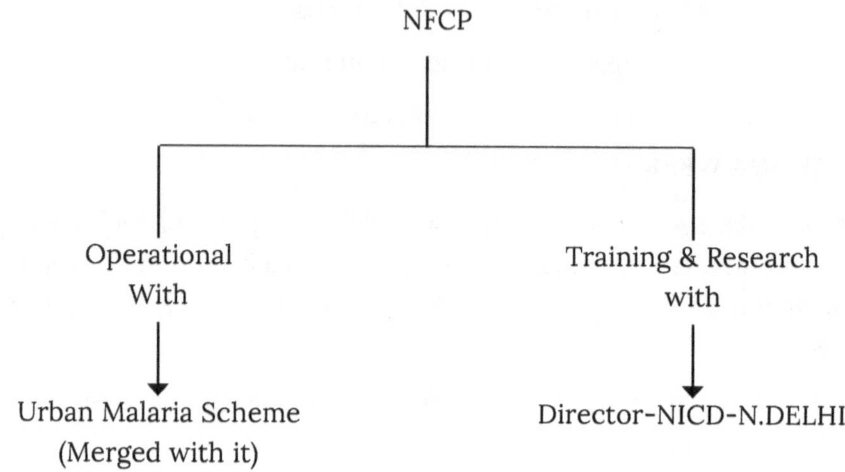

Activities under NFCP:

1. Survey in unserveyed area

2. Control in urban areas through–

    i.   Recurrent antiviral method

    ii. Anti parasitic methods

Horizontal Approach:

Utilized in coordination with "Primary Health Care System" & taking "village health guides" and "Local community participation"

Training: At (i) Regional Filaria Training & Research centre- Calicut (Kerala).

(ii) Regional Filaria Training & Research centre- Rajamundry (A.P.).

(iii) Regional Filaria Training & Research centre- Varanasi (U.P.).

Under NICD – (National Institute of Comm. Disease) and 12 HQ's Bureaus at state level.

SSB Level: Participates in community related Filarial Control programme.

3.2 (f)(ii) (3) NATIONAL LEPROSY "ERADICATION" PROGRAMME (NLEP)

The NLCP (National Leprosy Control Programme) has been into being since 1955.

It is a centrally aided programme to achieve – (11, 12)

    i   Early detection of cases and

    ii   DDS (Dapsone) chemo therapy to control leprosy

NLEP was initially in its infant and childhood stage and as such the growth of the programme was very slow for mostly two decades.

This programme gained speed with fourth "Five year programme" when it was made a centrally sponsored programme.

A working group was formed in 1980 which submitted its report in 1982 and recommended the following-

    i   MDT- Multi drug therapy

    ii   Reduction in quantum of infection &

    iii   Breaking the chain of transmission of disease.

In 1983, NLCP was redesignated as NLEP so as to eradicate it completely. Strategy :

The specific strategy is based on the following-

1. Early Detection of cases-

   - a) Population survey.

2. School survey.

3. Contact examination.

4. Voluntary referral.

5. Short term MDT.

6. Health education &

7. Rehabilitation activities.

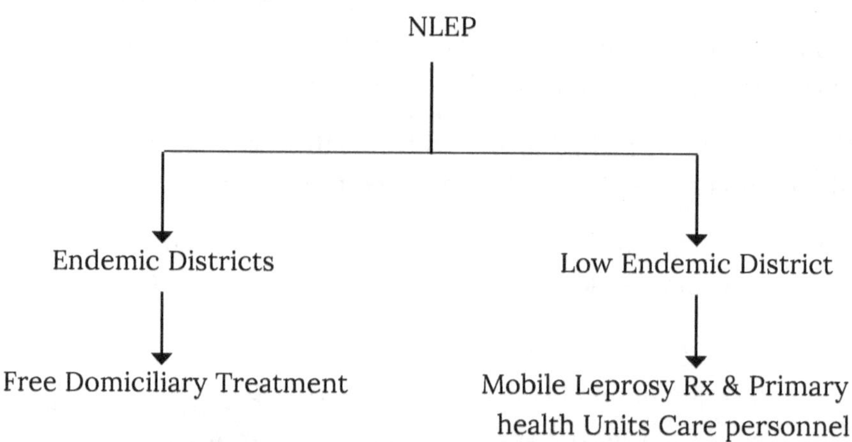

Infrastructure :

The infrastructure as envisaged by the NLEP is adhered to, which can be utilized by the SSB Para Military Staff also to come to a specific data related with leprosy patients in its/his area of operation .

Research into basic problems of leprosy is also important which is carried out by the Government Sector, via The Central Trauma Institute of Leprosy at Agra, The central Leprosy Teaching and

Training Institute at Chingelpur , Chennai & supported by Regional Training and Referral Institutes of ASKA (Orissa), Raipur (Chattisgarh) & Gouripur (West Bengal).

Foreign Assistance:

Considerable foreign assistances come (13, 14) especially from SIDA, WHO, UNICEF. Presently about 150 voluntary organizations are involved in anti leprosy activities besides the Government of India in its different forms.

Scenario at SSB Health Services:

SSB being on the Indo Nepal Border can give a good input to the central Government especially in the DARJEELING district, SILIGURI township & NAXALBARI area which are falling in its working zone. Health services are -as such- required to be augmented and the services of Para Medical Staff trained in such demographic data collection can be utilized for national redressal of leprosy.

3.2 (f)(ii) (4) NATIONAL TUBERCULOSIS PROGRAMME (NTP):

The National tuberculosis Programme has been in Operation since 1962.

Objectives:

a) Long term objective: Reduce TB in such a way that –

    i. One case infects less than one new person annually.

    ii. Prevalence below 14 years of age is brought down to < 1% against 30% at present.

b)   Operational/short term objective:

      i.   Detect maximum no. of TB cases and treat them effectively.

      ii.   Vaccinate new borne and infants with BCG in an integrated manner through all existing health institutions.

NTP operates thro District TB programme (DTP). Over 600 TB clinics have been set up out of which 390 have been up graded as District TB centre (DTC).

It was evolved by National TB institute, Bangalore & accepted by Government of India in 1962. Another important action (15) that came up was "BCG Vaccination" under National Immunization Programme, with the motive to protect all children by 1990.

NTP is a central programme with twin sharing (16) basis between the state and the centre.

Short term chemotherapy has been introduced as such 292 districts have been covered so for and other districts are in the pipeline too.

Some international agencies too are involved in this work like WHO, World Bank etc.

REVISED NATIONAL TB CONTROL PROGRAMME (RNTCP):

WHO & World Bank and Government of India revised the NTP in 1992. The specific features of this strategy are –

1.   85% cure rate through supervised short course chemotherapy

2.   Augmentation of case finding through quality sputum microcopy- 70%cases to be detected.

3. Involve NGOs- Information, Education and Communication & improved operation research under the revised NTP, active cases and finding will not be pursued. Case finding will be passive. 3 sputum smear examination will be required, besides X-Ray units set up at different location.

All patients will be provided short course chemotherapy under supervision called – DOTS-DIRECTLY OBSERVED THERAPY- SHORT TERM.

As such it ensured high cure rates, Through-

i Appropriate Medical treatment

ii Supervision

iii Motivation

By both Para Medical & Non Para Medical Staff. Scenario At SSB Health Services :

A direct surveillance thro Para Medical Staff and Doctors can go a long way in establishing control of TBC in and around Indo Nepal Border and eradicating TBC.

3.2 (f)(ii) (5) DIARRHOEAL DISEASE CONTROL PROGRAMME;

The National Diarrhoeal disease control programme was started during 6th plan to bring down Diarrhoeal mortality.

It was intensified during the Seventh Plan so as to reduce mortality by 50% by the year 1990. (17, 18) The programme is integrated within

    i   Primary Health Care Level-

          At - Village

          Sub centre

          PHC levels

    ii   District Hospital level

    iii   Private practitioners are also involved in it.

Every village health guide is supplied 100 packets of ORS/year, besides 200 packets supplied to sub centres functioning under family welfare programme.

Home made fluids and continuous feeding during diarrhea and recognition of early signs of dehydration besides promoting breast feeding for the 1st 4 to 6 months of life, proper weaning, infant immunization especially against Measles, and prophylaxis against vitamin-A deficiency is very much emphasized.

In 1993 a training schedule was also started for doctors to treat ACUTE GASTROENTERITIS cases with emphasis on ORAL REHYDRATION TREATMENT (ORS).

Supply of ORS packets is also enhanced depending upon the requirements. The Scenario at SSB:

In the SSB set up where most of the time potable drinking water is not available especially on the Indo Nepal Border, DIARRHOEAL TREATMENT UNITS (DTU) are the order of the day and it should be recognized as important.

3.2 (f)(ii) (6) STD CONTROL PROGRAMME:

STD control programme is the prevention of ill health (19, 20). These interventions may have –

> i   a primary prevention focus,
>
> ii   a secondary prevention focus (21) (for minimizing the adverse affects of infection on health).

As a perquisite of the above, the control depends upon-

1.   Initial Planning

2.   Intervention strategies

3.   Support components

4.   Monitory and evaluation.

> 1.   Initial Planning: Depends upon-
>
> > i.   Problem definition –
> >
> > Should be defined in terms of-
> >
> > > a.   Prevalence &
> > >
> > > b.   Psychosocial consequences.
> >
> > ii.   Establishing priorities –
> >
> > Basis being- Age, sex, place of residence, occupation, drug addiction etc.
> >
> > iii.   Setting objectives –
> >
> > Objective must be-Unambiguous and quantifiable.
> >
> > iv.   Considering strategics – Intervention strategics should be utilized.

2. Intervention Strategics :

These include:

    i.   Case detection.

    ii.   Cluster testing.

    iii.   Case holding and treatment.

    iv.   Epidemiological treatment.

    v.   Personal prophylaxis.

    vi.   Health education.

3. Support Components:

They include-

    i.   STD clinic.

    ii.   Lab services.

    iii.   Primary Health Care.

    iv.   Information system.

    v.   Legislation.

    vi.   Social Welfare Measures.

4. Monitoring & Evaluation-

Monitoring of disease trends and evaluating programme activities are effective strategies for a particular setting (22)

Scenario At SSB:

The CPMF personnel are bound by duty to remain out from their family members for months together. Physical requirements being a natural phenomenon for all -as such chances of STD is quite prevalent which requires a four pronged strategy as mentioned above- to nullify it.

SSB health services can be utilized quite competently to quash and nullify the effects of the same.

3.2 (f)(ii) (7) NATIONAL PROGRAMME FOR CONTROL OF BLINDNESS:

Launched : 1976

Aim : To reduce blindness from 1.4% to 0.3 % by the year 2010 AD; besides providing comprehensive eye care through primary health care.

Apex Institution : Dr. Rajendra Prasad centre for ophthalmic sciences Under AIIMS is established as a centre for –

  a. Manpower development

  b. Research &

  c. Referral services

3.2 (f)(ii) (8) NATIONAL IODINE DEFICIENCY DISORDERS (IDA) CONTROL PROGRAMME:

The Iodine Deficiency Control Programme was based on "GOITRE CONTROL PROGRAMME" of 1962, but it has been found that the prevalence of disease is quite high even today since a failure has been seen mostly on operations and logistics.

Demand and supply pace has been quite tardy leading to a high incidence of "GOITRE" cases.(25) Little impact could be seen on the "GOITRE RELATED PROGRAMMES"- because of this. (23)

The Problem:

According to Indian Council of Medical Research,(ICMR) the problem is not restricted to the "GOITRE- BELT" but can be seen also in –

    i   Gujarat

    ii   Punjab

    iii   Maharashtra

    iv   Madhya Pradesh

    v   Andhra Pradesh &

    vi   Kerala.

The Iodine Deficiency Manifestations are not seen only to "ENDEMIC GOITRE"& "CREATINISM" but to a wider spectrum of disability which include the following-

    a)   Deaf-mutism

    b)   Mental Retardation

    c)   Decreased Motor Functions

    d)   Decreased Motor intellect.

To ward off the problems being faced a major national programme i.e., the IDD control Programme has been initiated nation wide, rather a specific use of Iodized salt is being promoted.

By the end of 8th Plan this programme was to be implemented.

The basic components of a national IDD programme are –

    a)   Use of Iodized salt in place of common salt

    b)   Monitoring

    c)   Surveillance

    d)   Manpower Training &

    e)   Mass Communication.

Out of 28 states- 26 states have stopped use of salt without iodized component in it. A project of UNICEF has started monitoring this programme especially in-

1.   Assam

2.   Uttar Pradesh

3.   Madhya Pradesh

4.   Himanchal Pradesh

Covering 5 districts in cash state for reducing "GOITRE" in the age group 10-14 years to less than 5%.   The basic aim of this national programme is to bring down the incidence below 10% by the year 2010 of IDD.

SCENARIO AT SSB:

Planning for Iodized salt can be taken over by the Sashastra Seema Bal Para Medical staff in their area of operation thereby helping achieve bringing down the national incidenc3e below 10 percent by the year 2010.

3.2 (f)(ii) (9) NATIONAL IMMUNISATION SCHEDULE (NIS):

The Extended Programme (24) of Immunization (EPI) by WHO in May 1974 was utilized for prevention of six vaccine (25) preventable diseases –

i   Diphtheria

ii   Whooping Cough

iii   Tetanus

iv   Polio

v   Tuberculosis &

vi   Measles.

The Indian version is in the memory of Smt. Indira Gandhi late Prime Minister of India. The NIS that is followed is as follows –

a)   For Infants –

   1.   At Birth - BCG & OPV –O dose (For Institutional deliveries)

   2.   At 6 weeks- BCG (If not given at birth)- DPT-1 & OPV-1

   3.   At 10 weeks- DPT-2 & OPV-2

   4.   At 14 weeks- DPT-3 & OPV-3

   5.   At 9 months – MEASLES.

b)   At 16-24 months-

   DPT & OPV

c)   At 5-6 years- DT

d)   At 10 & At 16 Years-

   T.T. -2nd dose at an interval of 1 month.

e)   For Pregnant Woman –

   i   Early pregnancy -TT-1/Booster

   ii   One month after- TT-1 & TT-2 ROLE OF SSB IN NIS:

SSB Medical services can play an active role to implement NIS in the border population especially on INB & IBB not only by the Para Medical Staff, but the local population can also be involved to cater to it. Presently Pulse Polio Immunization Programme (PPIP) is actively supervised by the Sashastra Seema BAL Medical Services.

3.2 (f) (ii) (10) NATIONAL FAMILY WELFARE PROGRAMME:

The family planning programme was initiated in 1952, but birth control clinics have been functioning since 1930.

Basically the "small family norm" was to be adopted and accordingly things have been going on (26, 27). The 42nd Amendment of the constitution has made "Population control & family planning" a concurrent subject, and this provision has been made effective from January 1977.

In 1982, the Health for all policy came into being which was to be implemented up to the year 2000 AD but unfortunately this has not been the case and it is still not yet completed (28).

The Govt. of India has recently evolved a more detailed & comprehensive population policy to promote family planning & welfare on a voluntary basis. This can be seen from the investment of O.1. Crore during the 1st plan to Rs. 6500 crore during the Eight plan.

As such, it is imperative that the National Family Welfare Programe be completed to the hilt. The Scenario at SSB:

On the Indo Nepal Border the border population can be taken care of by the SSB personnel & Para Medical Staff to train them in birth Control clinics, methods, AIDS prevention and other health hazards of national importance complacency in tackling such problems can lead to further disaster in managing the health problems, as such training with regular work shops is the most important

factor that should be taken care. Provision for distribution of free condoms to the SSB personnel and the border population- can go a long way in completing this task to a satisfactory level.

3.2 (f) (ii) (11)   NATIONAL WATER SUPPLY & SANITATION PROGRAMME:

The National water supply and sanitation programme was started in 1954 for the benefit of both urban & rural population of the entire country (29, 30). "The accelerated Rural water supply programme" was commenced in 1972. The Central Govt. is identifying "problem villages" to assist the rural population.

A "Problem village" is defined as a village where no source of safe drinking water is available within a distance of 1.6 Kms or where water is available at a depth of more than 15 meters or where water source has excess salinity, iron, fluorides and other toxic elements or where water is exposed to "Cholera"& Guinea worm."

The Government of India launched "The International Drinking Water Supply & Sanitation Decade" in 1981.

The targets are –   (1)   100% for water < Urban Rural

(2)   80% for urban sanitation &

(3)   25% for rural sanitation.

The Scenario near SSB:

Since, about eighty percent of the deployment of SSB is on the Indo Nepal Border and Indo Bhutan Border which is basically village population and that too with rural background of the border villages – it can be emphasized with specifications that the SSB Health Services can take up the task of Rural Sanitation in a composite manner.

Specifications may be provided for the same and accordingly the Para Medical Staff can be provided with this responsibility to implement some of the water supply and sanitation programmes.

A total outlay of Rs 16711.03 crores were made during the Eighth Five Year Plan for this programme. Fund provisions can be made for the same, accordingly.

3.2 (f) (ii) (12)   GUINEA WORM ERADICATION PROGRAMME (GEP):

GEP was established during 1983-84. It was established without having a separate tactical organization.

Safe Drinking Water resources under the countries five year plans will look into the matter. As a matter of fact, it is quite important to eradicate Guinea Worm (31) just like poverty removal and it all is a matter of water treatment & training of the villager and people living there.

Performance appraised of the programme was made in 1985. In 1991 six states of India were endemically affected with 1906 villages in all being affected.

During this period Tamil Nadu worked open various anti - guinea worm measures and cases were not found after 1981.

The strategics involved in Guinea Worm eradication is multifold and the specific approaches are as follows –

- a) Provisions for Drinking Water on a priority basis to villages with endemicity.
- b) Vector Control with ABATE (TEMEPHOS) with a concentration of 1mg/lit.
- c) Health education.
- d) Personal prophylaxis-

  i.e. (i) Boiling of Drinking Water

  (ii) Sieving of unprotected water.

A few others are

e)   Nylon Mesh Filters

f)   Active Surveillances .

Scenario at SSB:

An important problem that the border population faces besides the villagers on the Indo Nepal Border is the Guinea Worm infestation. Since, the process of Health Education is a continuous process, personnel prophylaxis and Active surveillance is called for.

Work on control of the water sources by the SSB personnel by the use of Nylon Mesh Filter, Active surveillance, personnel prophylaxis, Health education by the Para Medical Staff and Doctors is called for with the active support of the administration. SSB can play its role in implementing this programme of national importance.

3.2 (f) (ii) (13)   MINIMUM NEEDS PROGRAMME (MNP):

MNP was introduced in the first year of the Five Year Plan (1974-78).

Basic Aim: The basic aim is to provide certain basic minimum needs and improve the living standards of the people.

The components included are -

a)   Rural Health.

b)   Rural water supply.

c)   Rural Electrification.

d)   Elementary education.

e)   Adult education.

f)   Nutrition.

g)   Improve urban slums.

h)   House for landless labourers.

A total of Rs. 2253.38 crores has been made in the 8th Five Year Plan as against Rs. 1063.35 crores in the 7th Plan for MNP in the state sector (32).

SCENARIO At SSB:

Rural areas on the Indo Nepal Border are covered (33) up to a range of 5 kms and besides developing nutritional packages- rural health, water supply, adult education and elementary education can be provided by the SSB personnel and Para Medical staff. It is only a matter of programme implementation

(34) that is required. Rural health & Elementary education is already being carried out since long. It is a factor related with guiding the SSB personnel to this line of thinking and thus providing the cutting edge to the rural population to work on such a line of thinking.

3.2 (f) (ii) (14) NATIONAL DIABETES CONTROL PROGRAMME (NDCP) :

OBJECTIVES :

The main objective are-

i	Identification of high risk subjects.
ii	Impart appropriate Health Education.
iii	Early diagnosis and management of cases.
iv	Prevention, arrest or slowing of Acute Metabolic process.
v	Slowing chronic cardio- Vascular- Renal complications, of the disease.

Control Focus :

SCENARIO AT SSB :

At   (i)   Sub centre level.

        (ii)   PHC level.

        (iiI) Dist Hospital level.

The two acute problems being faced in the SSB set up are-

        a)   Diabetes with obesity.

        b)   Hypertension.

Obesity and over weight with chronic indulgence in drinking episodes are almost the order of the day, besides leading to Hypertension.

As such the work of the Doctors and Para Medical Staff manifold and the importance there by of "National Diabetes Control Programme" comes into play what with the number of diabetes and hypertension cases increasing by the day.

3.2 (f) (ii) (15)   KALA AZAR CONTROL PROGRAMME:

Kala Azar is a serious public health hazard in -

        i   Bihar and

        ii   West Bengal

A total No. of 77101 cases were reported in 1992 with 1419 deaths, but this trend was arrested in 1993.

The Control Measures:

        i   Interruption of transmission for reducing vector population by undertaking indoor residual insecticide spray- twice annually.

ii   Early diagnosis.

iii   Complete treatment.

iv   Health education for community awareness.

Earlier the fund was being provided from the Government of India through NMEP budget provisions but –since 1992-93- Rs. 20.00 crores were provided against Annual plan outlay. The SSB Scenario:

SSB personnel are deployed on the Indo Nepal Border of more than 750 kms- out of which a few hundred kms are on Bihar and West Bengal borders-which are highly infested with Kala-Azar-especially prevalent during and after the monsoon season- when there is devastation by floods and later on- because of stagnant water.

To nullify the effects of Kala Azar the work related with such experiences on the Indo Nepal Border especially that of the SSB personnel required training and awareness regarding the disease and how it is caused. SSB Para Medical Staff can lend an active support to eradicate Kala Azar especially in Bihar and West Bengal. Accordingly policy decisions can be framed to ward of its menace.

3.2 (f) (ii) (16)   NATIONAL MENTAL HEALTH PROGRAMME (NMHP):

NMHP was launched during the seventh five year plan so as to achieve mental stability for the community at work and under privileged section of the population, (35) and the Geriatric population which suffers the most because of the mental and physical problems associated with old age (36).

A national advisory committee has been set up under the chairmanship of – Secretary, Ministry of H & F W for its effective implementation.

Scenario at SSB:

The working in the SSB or for that matter- any Para Military Force- is quite taxing what with emergency conditions arising every now and then, leading to problems related with leave etc. As such attending to family problems also gets hampered.

All these problems lead to development of Psychiatric problems on the part of SSB/force personnel thereby requiring mental mapping and enquiring what exactly is happening to the person concerned.

The work of the Doctors and Para Medical Staff- thus, is pronounced to know why this is happening?

Enquiry related with all these are thus, important to come to a conclusion and finally to a diagnosis related with the mental condition of the SSB personnel. This will finally lead to an exact treatment of the person.

3.2 (f) (ii) (17)   NATIONAL CANCER CONTROL PROGRAMME:

About 0.6 million cases are detected every year in relation to cancer cases.

Every Detection and alleviation of Sign/Symptoms (S/S) is the cornerstone of cancer the ropy. The following schemes have been initiated since 1990-91 –

1.   Scheme for District Projects –

    i   Preventive health education.

    ii   Early detection, and

    iii   Pain relief measures.

2.   Development of oncology wings in Medical Colleges/Hospitals.

Financial assistance unto Rs. 1 crore is provided to the concerned state Govt.for the purchase of equipments which includes one cobalt unit.

3.   Scheme for financial assistance to voluntary organizations.

An assistance of Rs. 5 lacs is provided to registered voluntary organizations recommended by state Government for undertaking health education and early detection of cancer.

Status at SSB:

At least the early detection at the deployment level- by the help of Para Medical Staff is called for. Surveillance of the village population is called for-in this regard.

Cirrhosis of liver, especially because of drinking binge- can be detected early- and treatment started accordingly.

3.2 (f) (ii) (18)   NATIONAL AIDS CONTROL PROGRAMME:

The National AIDS Control Programme was initiated in 1987 in India.

In 1991, a strategic plan for prevention and control of AIDS was developed. It was helped by WHO & World Bank and implemented in 1992 (37). The Ministry of health and family welfare has set up a National AIDS Control Organization (NACO) to implement and closely monitor the various components of the programme.

The national strategy is based on the following components –

1.   Establishment of Surveillance Centres.

2.   Identification of High Risk groups and screening.

3.   Issuing specific guidelines for management of detected cases and follow up.

4.   Formulating guidelines for blood banks.

5.   Blood product manufactures.

6.   Blood Donors.

7.   Dialysis units.

8.   Information, education & communication, activities by involving

- Mass Media

- Research

- Reduction of Stigma & social impact of the disease.

9.   Control of STD &

10. Condom programme.

At present 40 centres are conducting (38) Sentinel Surveillance leading to a –

i   Surveillance of Population Attending OPD of hospitals (Medical, Surgical, STD, antenatal & blood banks).

ii   Hospital based study to obtain data on prevalence of HIV infection in persons suffering from Tuberculosis & Leprosy.

Community based surveys for HIV infection (39). Investigations :

Early diagnosis and treatment of STD is a recognized procedure and strategy to control spread of HIV infection, since STD infected people are more prone to HIV infections.

The STD control provided recently are-

1. 5 Regional STD Reference centres in -

    - Delhi,

    - Chennai,

    - Hyderabad,

    - Nagpur &

    - Calcutta.

The Skin -Leprosy – STD clinics in Medical Colleges and in some district and Taluka Hospitals have been merged with AIDS control programme.

In recognition of the fact that some people have multiple sex partners and engage in sexual behavior which puts them at risk of acquiring STD/HIV, the Government of India strongly supports the promotion of good quality low cost condoms.

Scenario AT SSB:

Recently it has been observed that the SSB personnel who have been posted on the border with active duty have been approached with HIV infected girls so that the anti-national activities being propagated by the ISI agents and the Maoists reaches to the hilt and young boys and girls get infected with the dreaded virus. This will finish off both the youth and their reputation in the society. As such the work of the Para Medical Staff is quite important in this context and has to be implemented with the help of the Doctors and Administrators- both.

HIV/AIDS control programme is now of prime importance and as such VOLUNTARY, CONFIDENTIAL, COUNCELLING & TESTING (VCCT) CENTRES have come into force in the SSB-thereby- the importance of solving such a problem has gained in importance which will become quite forceful in the near future.

3.2 (f) (ii) (19) TWENTY POINT PROGRAMME-

Besides the five year plan and programme, in 1975 the 20 points programme was initiated to augment the following activities-

"Eradication of Poverty, Reducing inequalities, removing social and Economic inequalities and improving the quality of life"-is the basic theme of this twenty point programme.

The following points are directly or indirectly involved in the development of health for all and as such they are-

- Point 1. Attack on rural poverty.
- Point 7. Clean drinking water.
- Point 8. Health for all.
- Point 9. Two children Norm.
- Point 10. Expansion of education.
- Point 14. Housing for people.
- Point 15. Improvement of slums.
- Point 17. Protection of the environment.

All this was stated in 1986 on August 20. Scenario at SSB:

As per the existing situation in the SSB set up it has been found that Point No. 7, 8, 9, 10 & 17 are followed more or less and it is important to note- at this juncture that -Clean drinking water, Health or all. Two children Norm, Expansion of Education and protection of Environment- respectively-are important factors that are being taken care of and can be emphasized further with passage of time with the help of Para Medical Staff and Doctors of the department.

3.2 (f) (ii) (20) CHILD SURVIVAL AND SAFE MOTHERHOOD PROGRAMME:

The importance of the health of "Mother & Child" is emphasized in such a manner that you will find 9 out of 17 goals listed in the National Health Policy (1983) related to maternal and child health (40).With effect from August 1992 the programme named "Child Survival & Safe Motherhood"(CSSM) programme is being implemented with financial assistance from World Bank and UNICEF (41).

The objectives:

1.   (a) Sustain & Strengthen the ongoing universal Immunization Programme.

   (b) Continuous ORAL REHYDRATION THERAPY (ORT) Programme for children below 5 years.

   (c) Protecting from ARDS/infection for children below 5 years of age.

2.   (a) Prophylactic scheme to control blindness due to deficiency of Vitamin-A for children less than or equal to 3 years age.

   (b) Nutritional scheme against Anemia amongst Pregnant & Lactating (P&L) mothers, as well as children upto 5 years of age- through administration of Iron and Folic Acid tablets.

3.   (a) Improving new born care and mother care at the community level.

The Scenario in SSB:

Universal Immunization Programme (UIP) is a continuous programme and Pulse Polio Immunization Programme (PPIP) is being implemented throughout the SSB set up in collaboration with Medical colleges and Hospitals and the Doctors and Para Medical Staff of the SSB set up.

3.2(f) (iii)   CONCLUSIONS:

Health policy documents as envisioned above are quite important for the development of the country as well as the SSB as a whole. Thus, work has to be supplemented for health services in the light of the above facts.

Chapter 4
Methodology

4.1 INTRODUCTION:

This Chapter presents the methodology comprising the Questionnaire method & Situational analysis comprising the External Environment Analysis, The Existing Health care System, The Internal Environment Analysis.

The Research Design (Methodology) used in this study has been extensively described in this Chapter. It studies the development of Questionnaires, Sampling Method & Selection of targeted Staff and Administration of Questionnaires on both the SSB Personnel and External Beneficiaries who take the benefit & help of SSB Health Services.

The Research Design is important in the knowhow regarding "Planning & Structure of Issue" to be investigated.

Research Design depicts the frame work of the relationship of the variables involved in the study & systematic investigations to obtain solid inferences for the benefit of the research being carried out.

4.2 RESEARCH DESIGN PROCESS:

The Research Design Process that has been exclusive to the strategic Management of SSBHS can be summarized as follows: -

RESEARCH DESIGN
(TYPE, PURPOSE)

DEVELOPMENT/SELECTION OF QUESTIONNARIE
{PURPOSE, RELEVENCE, PRETESTING}

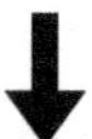

SAMPLE DESIGN
{SAMPLING FRAME, SAMPLING METHOD}

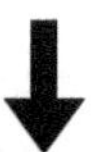

COLLECTION OF DATA

{PERSONAL INTERVIEW, ADMINISTRATING QUESTIONNAIRE & CONCEPT CLASSES FOR FAMILIARIZATION & SITUATIONAL ANALYSIS COMPRISING THE EXTERNAL ENVIRONMENT ANALYSIS, THE EXISTING HEALTH CARE SYSTEM, THE INTERNAL ENVIRONMENT ANALYSIS.}

ANALYSIS OF DATA

{Includes RESULTS *of* QUESTIONNAIRE, SITUATIONAL ANALYSIS COMPRISING THE EXTERNAL ENVIRONMENT ANALYSIS, THE EXISTING HEALTH CARE SYSTEM, THE INTERNAL ENVIRONMENT ANALYSIS *&* SWOT *Analysis &* DISCUSSIONs *thereof}*

ANALYSIS OF DATA

{Includes RESULTS *of* QUESTIONNAIRE, SITUATIONAL ANALYSIS COMPRISING THE EXTERNAL ENVIRONMENT ANALYSIS, THE EXISTING HEALTH CARE SYSTEM, THE INTERNAL ENVIRONMENT ANALYSIS *&* SWOT *Analysis &* DISCUSSIONs *thereof}*

Figure 4.1 – Research Design Process

Thus, the Research Design Process involves instrument Selection, Data Collection & Analysis which has been depicted as above.

The subsequent information about each step is depicted in this Chapter step by step.

4.3 RESEARCH DESIGN:

Research Design is defined as "the arrangement of conditions for collection & analysis of data in a manner that aims to combine relevance to Research purpose with Economy in procedure." {Kothari – 1999}

Research Design should have a "clear statement of the Research problem, procedures & techniques for gathering information, the population to be studied & the methods used in processing & analyzing data."

As such, the essential features of a Research Design should contain –

    i   On the basis of the Research question there should be an activity & time based plan or strategy.

    ii   A frame work for specifying the relationships among the study's variables with a specific (Procedural) outline for each and every activity.

Different authors propose different types of Research Design. According to Bryman & Bell (2006) Research Design can have- Experimental Design, Cross Sectional Design, Longitudinal Design, Cross Study Design and Comparative Design. According to Zikmund (2005) & Cooper & Schindler (2007) research design can be Exploratory & Descriptive & Causal, Whereas Kothari (1999) suggests the design to be Exploratory, Descriptive and diagnostic, Hypothesis testing types.

In case of the study for Sashatra Seema Bal, a strategic plan for health services the Research Design that has been propose will incorporate the following:

Exploratory type in nature:

Exploratory Research targets at obtaining complete & accurate information with multiple provisions for safeguarding against prejudices & biases and even prior perceptions which helps in the complete reliability of the data.

A survey research has been conducted which comprises "a cross sectional design" relating to data being collected by questionnaire method & structured interview for "SSB personnel" & "External

Beneficiaries" with different variables to detect patterns of association (Bryman & Bell, 2006).

A cross sectional design examination of relationships between variables helps in such a way that the margin of manipulation by the researcher becomes minimal. Here, in the cross sectional design examination research data on the variables of interest are collected simultaneously.

Hypothesis based research has also been employed to test the Hypothesis of causal relationships (cause & effect) between variables. These studies require reliability. Multiple Hypothetical statements have been incorporated in this study but have been statistically tested & variables and found to be spot on.

TABLE 4.1 POSITIONING OF RESEARCH DESIGN

SL. NO.	CATEGORY	DESCRIPTOR
1	Degree of Crystallization of the Research.	Formal Study
2	Data Collection Method.	Communication Study.
3	Power of Researches to produce effects in the variables.	Ex post facto..
4	Purpose of study.	Strategically manage SSB Health Services.
5	The time dimension	Cross sectional.
6	Scope.	Statistical.
7	Research Environment.	Field setting.

According to the table 4.1 it can be safely prescribed that the strategic plan for SSB Health Services is a formal study with communication process type of data collection method. It tests the hypothesis or answers the research question posed. The researchers questions the subjects and collects their responses besides administering the instrument personally to the SSB personnel and external beneficiaries.

Further, the study is a cross sectional field setting type of study. Cross sectional study is carried out only once and represents a snap shot at one point in time.

The Research has been carried out in field settings especially with the Indo-Nepal Border of Sikkim, W. Bengal and Bihar with special emphasis on BOPs (Border Observation Posts), Coys (Companies) & Battalions.

4.4 SELECTION OF QUESTIONNAIRE:

What is the purpose?

The purposes of questionnaires are to collect data efficiently when the researcher knows how to measure the variables of interest.

A questionnaire is a set of written questions where the responders record their answers, usually having closely defined alternatives. Research bias can be minimized if the awarding of the questions, general appearance of questionnaire and planning of issues of how the variables will be categorized scaled and coded after the receipt of response.

A through measurement analysis on survey instrument is a must during this survey through questionnaires. This analysis helps quantify that the results are accurate measurements and results are believable.

What is the relevance?

The selection of questionnaire should be reliable and to the paint, short and simple (Kothari, 1999), should proceed in a logical sequence with easier questions at the start and then the more difficult ones. Term based questions should be avoided especially technical in nature. As such the questionnaire was selected by the much acclaimed performance discrepancy indicator that was provided by Dr. Y. K. Gupta, (I/P- Family and Health Welfare, Jammu) and Dr.

N. S. Gupta of IMPA, Jammu & Kashmir (Through, HIPA, Gurgaon-Exhibit I & Exhibit II).

The questionnaire so provided was implemented on both the SSB personnel and external beneficiaries outside the ambit of SSB but within 15 Kms. Of area of operation of SSB.

4.4.1 COMPILATION OF QUESTIONNAIRES:

The question to be administered relates to Performance Discrepancy Indicator developed by Gupta & Gupta (1996) of H & FW – J & K and IMPA, J & K clubbed together with George and Shrivastava (of HIPA, April- 1996) for measurement of organizational climate.

A.   The areas of performance that were in the area of consideration were:

    i   Health Care Cost.

    ii   Quality.

    iii   Health Targets (HIV/AIDS, VCCT).

    iv   Essential Drugs.

    v   Transfer/Postings.

    vi   Absentism.

    vii   Compliance to service rules.

    viii Co-Ordinations.

    ix   Equipments.

    x   X-Ray films etc.

B.   The responses have been rated on a three point performance discrepancy indicator namely "O" meaning no problem, between" 20-30" means on organizational climate you can live with & "50" means serious problem.

C. **RAW SCORE:**

The raw score is divided from Zero (0) to Fifty (50) with a margin of five in between. The total of each response of all the fifteen questions is computed as the Raw Score.

D. **EFFECTIVE SCORE:**

The Raw Score for each item on the questionnaire is divided by ten (10) for recording the effective score.

E. **TEMPERATURE:**

The effective score represents the temperature of the Organization.

4.4.2 SELECTION WITH PDI QUESTIONNAIRE FOR SSB PERSONNEL:

In the strategic plan study for effective Health Services for SSB, the Performance Discrepancy Indicator has a role to play since the questionnaires were based on the goals and objectives selected for the SSB personnel. If any changes were required they were incorporated in the questionnaire and tested for biases if any and ruled out if per chance one crept in. A high score on any specific question reflects a high level of social & emotional competency, besides the relevance factor of that particular objective is also highlighted. Gupta & Gupta (IMPA- 1996) have reported that- PDI has a replicable factor structure i.e. the various scales on the PDI instrument correlate highly with comparable scales on the external beneficiaries. In this case both SSB Personnel and External Beneficiaries (EB) results correlate highly. The PDI has a built in correction factor that can adjust the scores automatically for self-report measures in that it reduced the distasting effects of bias based on social response and this has led to increasing the accuracy of the results so gathered. PDI also includes medical inventory that is utilized on a day to day basis and whether the misuse of equipments, drugs, X-Ray Films, reagents etc. is rampant or not- is also measured. Questions based on responsibility and compliance is also incorporated in the PDI. Data related with income, occupation and literacy levels of each responded has also been included. The data from SSB personnel has also been incorporated.

4.4.3 SELECTION OF PDI QUESTIONNAIRE FOR EXTERNAL BENEFICIALITIES OUT SIDE THE AMBIT OF SSB BUT- WITHIN THE RANGE OF WORKING OF SSB.

The Performance Discrepancy Indicator for External Beneficiaries to measure effectiveness of SSB Health Services on the external environment was entrusted for research through Gupta & Gupta (1996 & 2006-2008) of IMPA & H & FW- JMCH.

The PDI measured Interpersonal Relationship, adaptability, Stress Management & Equipment Management & Morale of Health Care Worker (HCW).

The Interpersonal relationship PDI measures Self Awareness, Self Actualization, & Independence from SSB influence, the ability to view oneself positively besides the ability to assert one self. The second, i.e. The Interpersonal Relationship empathies with social responsibility. The third, i.e. Stress Management-PDI measures skills like Stress Tolerance & Impulse Control. The four, i.e. Adaptability PDI studies Flexibility, Problem Solving & Reality Testing. The fifth, that is Equipment Management studies whether the equipments have been maintained properly or not including dispension of drugs etc,.Finally, the Morale of HCW is studied through the PDI which includes working without resentment i.e. being happy and optimistic.

The responses are rated on a scale of (i) zero (0) being no problem, (ii) Twenty- five to Thirty-five (25-35) being an organizational climate where you can live & work happily and (iii) fifty (50) being Serious Problem.

4.4.4 PRE-TESTING:

The basic purpose of pretesting are:

- a) Select and establish the appropriate response.
- b) To see that the Questions in the questionnaire can be easily understood.
- c) To find out whether the measuring instrument is effective or otherwise.

The Pre-Testing was carried out in two stages.

In the first stage the draft of the questionnaire was provided to two brilliant academicians who were requested to evaluate the items from the standpoint of specificity & clarity of construction. Gupta & Gupta of IMPA & HIPA did the check and provided the necessary imports for carrying out the questionnaire.

In the second pretesting the questionnaire was given to SSB personnel and external beneficiaries outside the ambit of SSB and were asked to check and complete the questionnaire and spell out any suggestions and weed out any irrelevant questions related with Health & Health Services. This pretesting was carried out by Officers/Officials of different branches amounting to about twenty (2 each from different branch) & from people of different walks of life outside the ambit of SSB.

This led to a review of the questionnaire based on expects comments and thereby modifying the questions in such a way that the exquisite research instrument became specific & up to the mark in Its effectiveness.

It was further found, during pretesting that the SSB personnel took about 15-20 mts. while external beneficiaries took about 10-15 mts. to do the same exercise.

4.5.1 SAMPLING FRAME:

A Sampling Frame is generally closely related to the population in question. In this regard the population in question is the SSB personnel & external beneficiaries outside SSB.

It is a list of elements (types of personnel from SSB & outside it) from which generally the sample is drawn (coupes & sentinels, 2007). As such the relation of sample for this strategic plan for effective Health Services for SSB is based on the following craiteratia:

i   SSB personnel belonging to an age group of 45-55 years were selected to participate.

ii   Family income & socio-economic status of the SSB personnel was also looked into.

iii   Permission was granted to administer the questionnaire in the SSB premises as well as at the residence of external beneficiaries.

iv   Years of service was also mapped in detail which was between 15-20 years for the SSB personnel.

4.5.2 SAMPLING METHOD:

A sample is a specific part of a population, which is selected to obtain necessary information. (Cooper & Shindler, 2007). Thus, when a small group is taken as the representative of the whole, the study is called "Sampling Study". The whole group from which the sample has been drawn is technically known as "Universe" or "Population" and the group actually selected for study is known as sample.

Sampling Method can be classified as:

    i   Probability &

    ii   Non-Probability Sampling.

1.   **PROBABILITY SAMPLING:** Probability Sampling is based on the concept of RANDOMISATION OR RANDOM SELECTION.

It is a process of sampling where each and every element of the population has a Non-Zero chance of selection. This is a process where there is "PRECISION" in the estimates and is never haphazard or topsy-turvy.

2.   **NON-PROBABILITY SAMPLING:** It is a method which is carried out having a scheme or pattern in mind and depends upon the Whims & Fancy of the Researcher (i.e. subjective).Each member of the population does not get a chance for inclusion.

4.5.3 TYPE OF SAMPLING DESIGN:

Elemental Selection	Probability	Non-Probability
Unrestricted	Simple Random	Convenience
Restricted	Complex Random	Purposive Judgment Quota
	Systematic	Snowball
	Cluster	
	Stratified	
	Double	

Non-Probability, purposive quote sampling method was used for collection of data for SSB personnel. Purposive sampling includes obtaining necessary group from specific target groups.

This sampling is confined to certain types of people because of two reasons:

a) Conformity with some criteria set by the researcher. Quota sampling (E.g. for Scheduled Tribes (ST) Height (Ht) is set at 162.5 cms for Constables to be appointed to the SSB ranks.)

b) Some specific people have the information (Judgment Sampling). (E.g. Doctors who treat Psychiatric patients.)

As such, based on some specific criteria set by the researcher "QUOTA SAMPLING" technique has been used in this research.

This method of sampling, i.e. Quota sampling helps in adequately representing certain groups in the study and throughout the length of the study (SEKARAM, 2007). A quota is fixed for each Sub-group based on the total number of each group in the population. Quota sampling is stratified groups from which subjects are selected randomly.

4.5.4 SAMPLE OF SSB PERSONNEL:

SSB personnel working under Frontier Hqrs. SSB Patna were considered and the following criteria were considered. The no. of years in service, qualifications related with Post-Doctoral, Post Graduation, Under Graduation, Matriculation & Non-Matriculation Examinations conducted by different Boards of different states besides Secondary School Certificate Examination (SSCE) and Indian Central Board schools like Indian School Certificate examination (ICSE) & Central Board of Secondary Education (CBSE) were taken cognizance of. Personnel belonging to different states, religion and caste were also included in the study. Data of SSB personnel in special areas on the border were also considered like Thakurganj and Kishanganj etc.

Summarizing, personnel different ethnic groups were considered. The various classifications included urban- rural personnel, residential- non-residential personnel, tribal- non-tribal SSB personnel.These personnel represent diverse socio-economic back ground characterized by upbringing of the SSB personnel in a rural urban area, with differing levels & Parental literacy, occupation and family income.Criteria based on SSB personnels characterstics:

CRITERIA	PARENT	LEVEL	CATEGORY
Literary	Father	1	Up to 10th st.
		2	Graduate
		3	PG/Prof. Edu.
	Mother	1	Up to 10th st.
		2	Graduate
		3	PG/Prof. Edu.
Occupation	Father	0	Father expired. Father in lowly job. Father in service.
		1	
		2	Father manages business. Father is professor.
		3	
		4	
	Mother	0	Mother expired. Mother in lowly job. Mother in service.
		1	
		2	Mother manage business
		3	Mother is professor.
		4	
Family income	Father	1	Up to 1,00000 (LIG)
		2	Up to 1 lack – 5 lack (MIG)
		3	> 5 lack (HIG)

Table-4.5.4.SAMPLE OF SSB PERSONNEL

Literacy, Occupation & Family Income is also considered for classification of student type. Based on the data, parental categorization is shown. Literacy & Occupation is also considered of each parent. Economics based on house hold income is also categorized. A "Purposive Quota Sampling" technique was used for the study and the questionnaire administered amongst the SSB personnel.

The stability & equivalence aspect of reliability was maintained during data collection procedure by administrating the questionnaire personally. Workshops & personal interviews too were considered personally ensuring the automaticity of data collection. SSB personnel, in exchange for their participation, were provided with confidential feed back reports on the results on each of the question.

4.5.5 SAMPLE OF EXTERNAL BENEFICIARIES:

The sample size was more or less same numbering 5100 from different areas of operation. Different beneficiaries were taken from different regions.

The data was collected from different circles, SHQ areas and area (near Kishanganj, Darjeeling district) to have a picture of the relevance of the questionnaire supplied for finding out the relevance of SSB Health Services.

4.5.5.1 CRITERIA FOR CLASSIFICATION OF EXTERNAL BENEFICIARIES

CRITERIATION	TYPE
Circle	Rimbik, Loleygaon, Thakurganj
Sub-Area	Darjeeling, Mirik, Thakurganj
Area	Darjeeling, Kishanganj

These beneficiaries represent diverse socio-economic back ground characterized by different food habits, upbringing, parental occupation & family income. The count of the external beneficiaries based on family income was also considered.

4.5.5.2 COLLECTION OF DATA:

A covering letter was sent to the different branch heads, which included general information about the research work & the instruction used for the study, confidentiality of the responses and request for returning the filled up questionnaire. Collection of data was done between March to October 2006. A workshop for the SSB personnel along with personnel interview for senior personnel was an added activity that was conducted.

4.5.5.3 WORKSHOP FOR SSB PERSONNEL:

A workshop is an educational seminar or a series of meetings emphasizing interaction & exchange of information among a usually small number of participants (According to the American Heritage Dictionary). Once, the authorities agreed the researcher conducted the test in their premises, while a workshop was conducted for the SSB personnel to explain the contents of the questionnaire. How the personnel listened and how much interest they took in the understanding of the questions was also observed?

4.5.5.4 PERSONNEL INTERVIEW:

Personnel Interview require a person known as an interviewer asking questions face to face with the other person or persons (Kothari, 1999).

It may be "Direct Personal Investigation" (DPI) or it may be an "Indirect oral Investigation" (DOI). DPI was conducted regarding the attitude & behavior of the SSB personnel & specific comments were noted by the senior officials.

4.5.5.5 ANALYSIS OF RESULTS & INTERPRETATIONS

The analysis of results and interpretation of the same was further carried out in the following sequence:

i   A comparison of Questionnaire results of SSB personnel with that of external beneficiaries.

ii   The External Environment Analysis, The Existing Health Care Analysis, The Internal Environment Analysis.

iii   A SWOT Analysis of major factors involved in the day to day working of the SSB Head Quarters.

Chapter 5
RESULTS & DISCUSSION

5.1 INTRODUCTION:

A detailed audit of the organization is needed to identify strengths, weaknesses, opportunities and threats and create a baseline. In this chapter, the results obtained by The Questionnaire method, The External Environment Analysis, The Existing Health Care Analysis, The Internal Environment Analysis, the Results of a SWOT Analysis are discussed in detail leading to the creation of a Strategic plan for SSB Health Services.

5.2 THE QUESTIONNAIRE METHOD:

During the study for developing a strategic plan for effective health services for SSB the following Methodology was followed -

(1) Direct – (a) Survey of personnel from Sashastra Seema Bal.

(b) Survey of beneficiaries outside the ambit of Sashastra Seema Bal.

5.2(1) (a) Survey of personnel from Sashastra Seema Bal:

(i) *Methodology:* A questionnaire was sent to the above mentioned SSB personnel who had to respond to fifteen parameters related with Medical services. Theses parameters are a checklist of performance discrepancy which has been incorporated in its present form to suit the necessity of Sashastra Seema Bal requirements. The basics have been provided by Dr. N.S. Gupta of IMPA, Jammu and Kashmir and Dr. Y.K. Gupta H&FW Jammu.

Summary of Results:

The Conclusions arrived at by the analysis of the checklist of performance discrepancy indicators provided the following results:-

Total No. of employees : 15,000

No. of respondents   : 344

Scale :   0 = No problem;   50 =   Serious problem; 25-35 = An organizational climate you can live with.

1.   Medical/Health care cost to the patients in the government health institutions has remained same/increasing in the last few years.

Scale		No. of Respondents	Percentage
a.	20	116	(34.45) = 34%
b.	25	118	(32.16) = 32%
c.	30	110	(33.39) = 33%

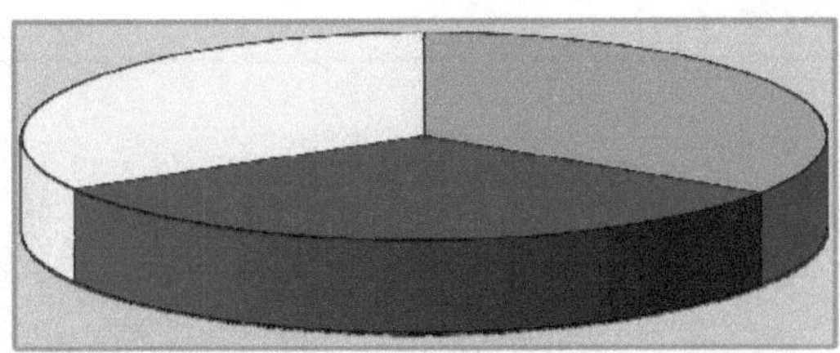

Yellow   = 33%

Violet   = 32%

Red   = 34%

2. Government health delivery system provides quality services as per the expectations of patients/clients.

a.	40	118	(34.60) = 35%
b.	30	110	(31.45) = 31%
c.	35	116	(33.95) = 34

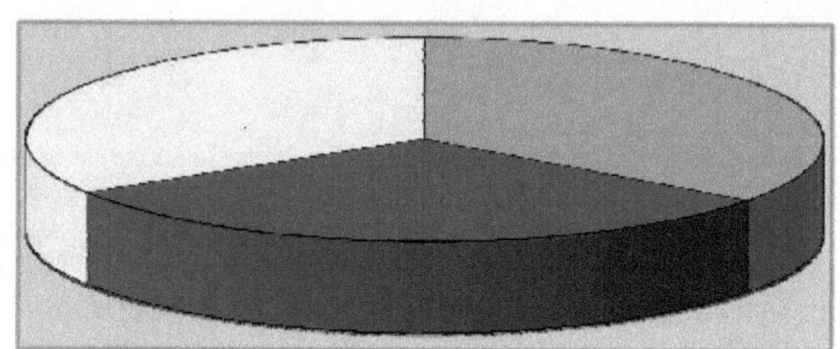

Yellow = 35%

Violet = 31%

Red = 34%

3. Targets of health programmes are being met

a.	20	120	36%
b.	40	110	30%
c.	25	114	34%

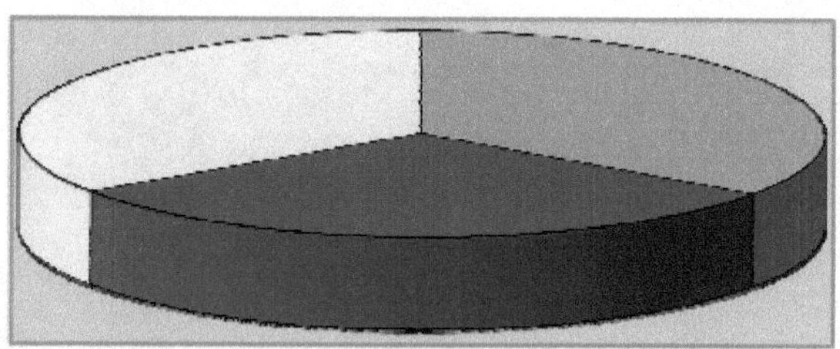

Yellow = 36%

Violet = 30%

Red = 34%

4. Patients/ clients complaints regarding poor functioning of govt. hospital/ health centers.

a.	40	110	32%
b.	45	92	28%
c.	20	142	40%

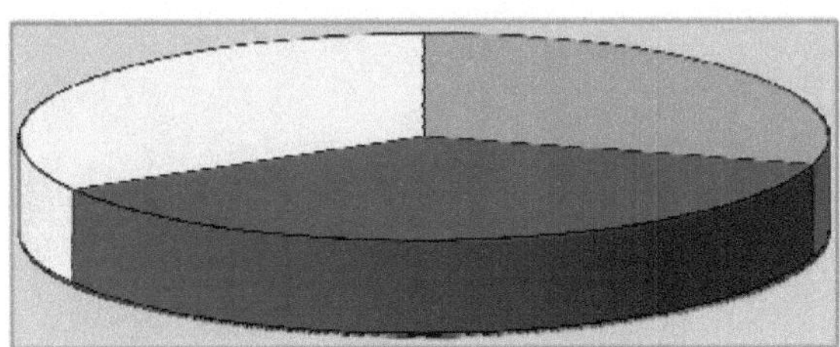

Yellow   = 32%

Violet   = 28%

Red   = 40%

5. Job functions of the team members are not evenly distributed

a.	30	110	30%
b.	35	92	32%
c.	40	142	38%

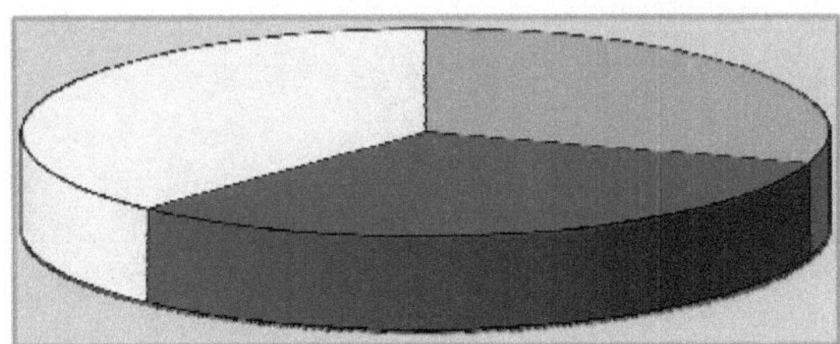

Yellow   = 30%

Violet   = 32%

Red   = 38%

6. Essential drugs in the government hospital/health centers are adequate

a.	25	130	36%
b.	35	140	40%
c.	45	74	24%

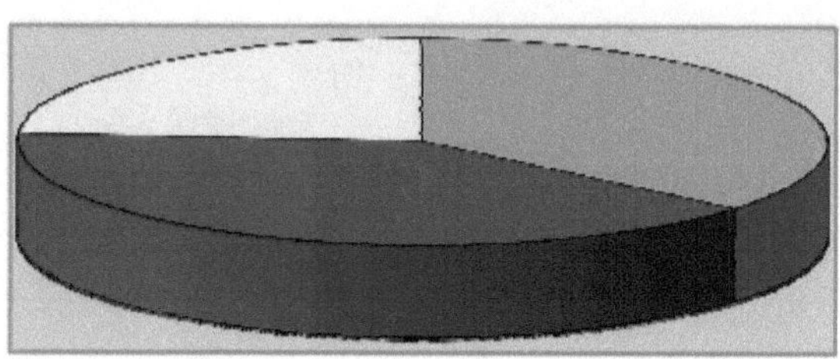

Yellow   = 36%

Violet   = 40%

Red   = 24%

7. Work load on HCW's is more than what can be handled

a.	30	130	40%
b.	40	140	34%
c.	35	74	26%

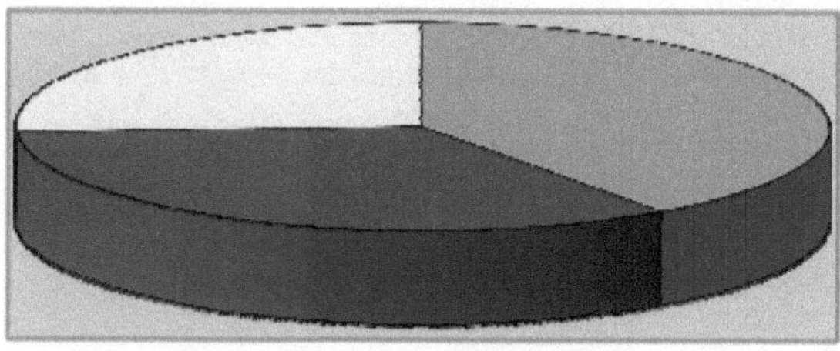

Yellow   = 40%

Violet   = 34%

Red   = 26%

8. Transfers/ postings are frequent and not based on any rationale

a.	20	110	34%
b.	45	92	26%
c.	40	142	40%

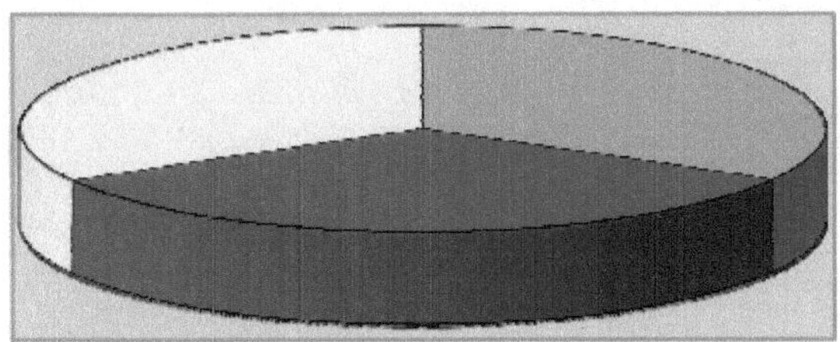

Yellow = 34%

Violet   = 26%

Red   = 40%

9. Absenteeism is common feature in the govt. health care delivery system

a.	20	110	32%
b.	30	92	28%
c.	35	142	40%

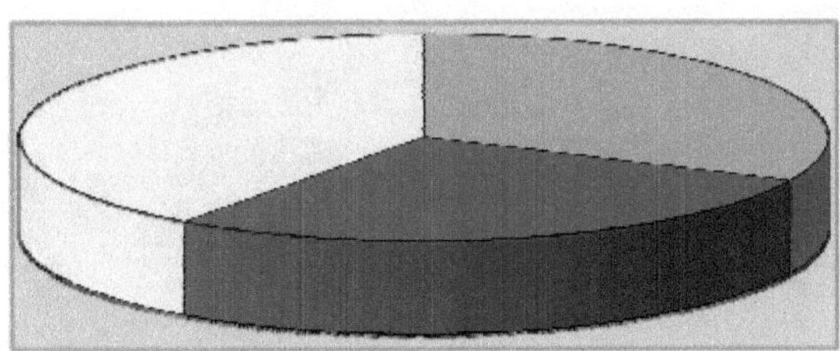

Yellow = 32%

Violet   = 28%

Red   = 40%

10.   Morale of HCW's is low, as compared to other govt. employees

a.	25	110	40%
b.	45	92	36%
c.	35	142	24%

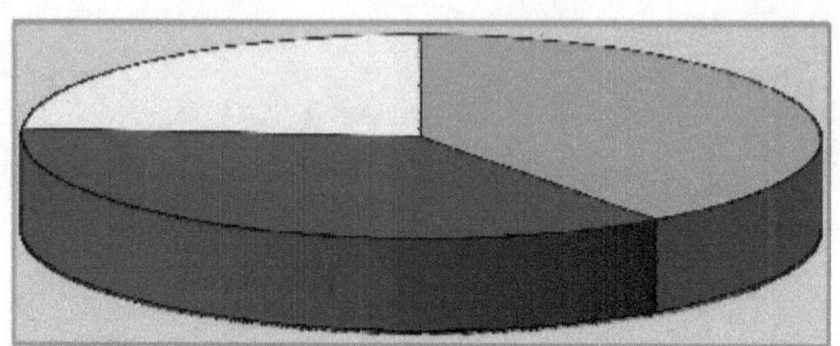

Yellow   = 24%

Violet   =36 %

Red   = 40%

11.   Inter-personal conflicts are common within the health team

a.	25	110	32%
b.	35	92	28%
c.	40	142	40%

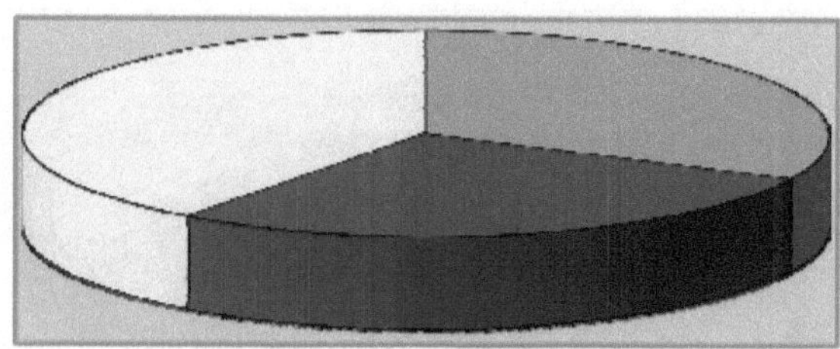

Yellow   = 40%

Violet   =28 %

Red   = 32%

12. Non – compliance with the superiors orders and service rules is common among HCW's

a.	30	130	38%
b.	40	140	40%
c.	35	74	22%

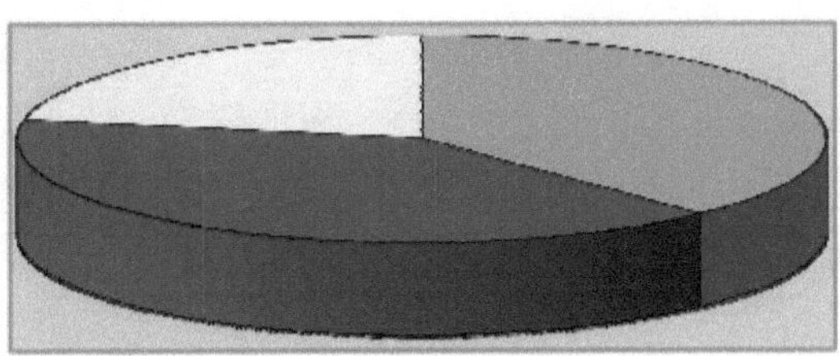

Yellow   = 22%

Violet   =40 %

Red   = 38%

13. Co- operation and co-ordination within the health team is low

a.	25	130	40%
b.	35	140	36%
c.	45	74	24%

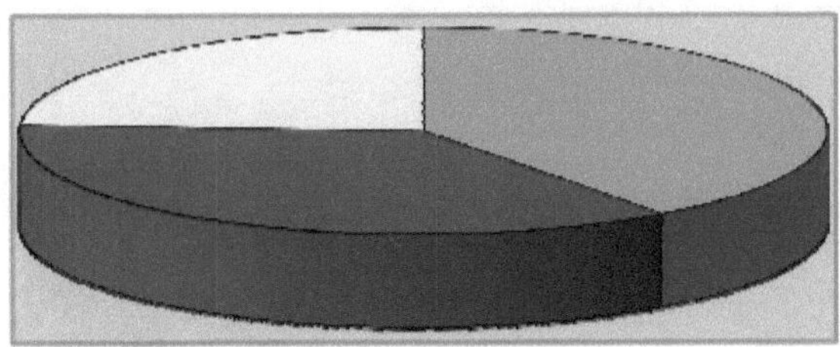

Yellow   = 24%

Violet   =36 %

Red   = 40%

14. Most of non-functional equipment in government health institutions requires minor repairs.

a.	20	130	38%
b.	35	140	40%
c.	40	74	22%

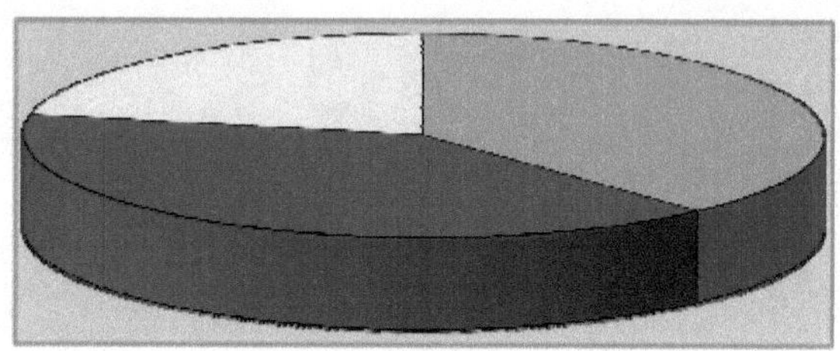

Yellow = 2%

Violet   =40 %

Red   = 38%

15. Misuse of equipment/ drugs X-Ray films/ reagents etc. is quite common

a.	30	130	36%
b.	45	140	40%
c.	25	74	24%

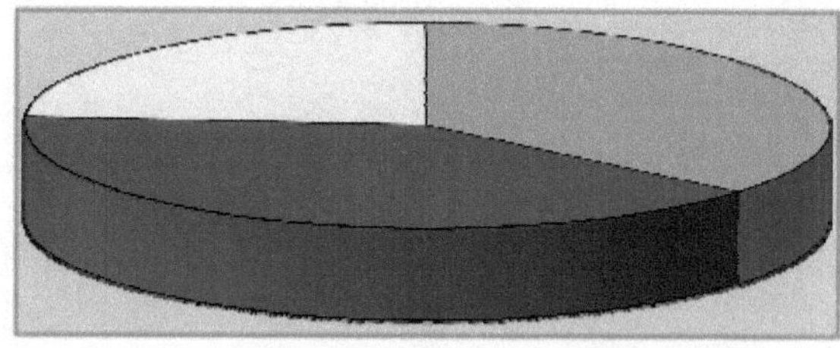

Yellow   = 24%

Violet   =40 %

Red   = 36%

(Exhibit No. 1]

The Measurement of Organizational Climate

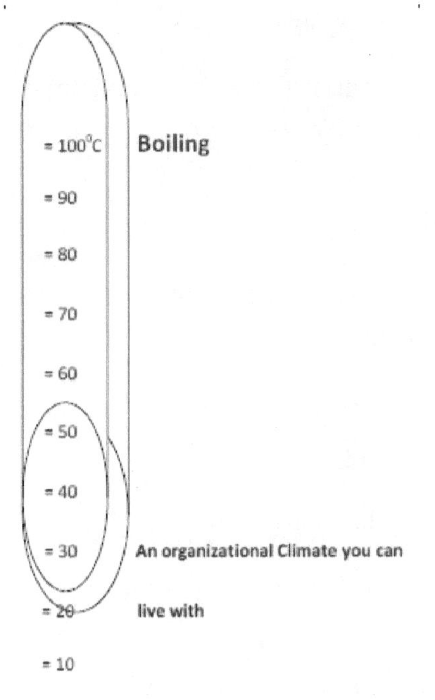

1. Areas of Performance
2. Health Care Cost.
3. Quality.
4. Health Targets.
5. Essential Drugs.
6. Transfer/Postings
7. Absenteeism.
8. Compliance to Service Rules.
9. Coordination.
10. Equipments
11. X-ray Film, etc. Ref. (2)

Ref. : Action Research & Planning for Decentralization. Editions : Dr. J. George & S. Srivastava, HIPA, April 1996.

Taking temperature of your organization.

(Effective score is taken from the performance Discrepancy Indicator vide Exhibit No. 2)

[Exhibit No.-2]

PERFORMANCE DISCREPANCY INDICATORS

Remember: 0 = no problem; 50 = serious problem

1. Medical/Health care cost to the patients in the government health institutions has remained same/ been increasing in the last few years.

    0   10   15   20   25   30   35   40   45   50   ....

2. Government health delivery system provides quality services as per the expectations of Patients/clients.

    0   10   15   20   25   30   35   40   45   50   ....

3. Targets of health programmes are being met

    0   10   15   20   25   30   35   40   45   50   ....

4. Patients/clients complaints regarding poor functioning of Govt. Hospitals health centers.

    0   10   15   20   25   30   35   40   45   50   ....

5. Job functions of the team members are not evenly distributed.

    0   10   15   20   25   30   35   40   45   50   ....

6. Essential drugs in the Govt. Hospital/health centers are adequate.

    0   10   15   20   25   30   35   40   45   50   ....

7. Workload on HCW's is more than what can be handled.

    0   10   15   20   25   30   35   40   45   50   ....

8. Transfers/postings are frequent and not based on any rationale

    0   10   15   20   25   30   35   40   45   50   ....

9.   Absenteeism is a common feature in the Govt. Health Care delivery system

    0   10   15   20   25   30   35   40   45   50   ....

10.   Morale of HCW's is low as compared to other Govt. employees.

    0   10   15   20   25   30   35   40   45   50   ....

11.   Interpersonal conflicts are common within the health team.

    0   10   15   20   25   30   35   40   45   50   ....

12.   Non compliance of services rule exists in health services.

    0   10   15   20   25   30   35   40   45   50   ....

13.   Improper coordination exists in the health team.

    0   10   15   20   25   30   35   40   45   50   ....

14.   Most of the equipment in Govt. Health institutions requires minor repairs.

    0   10   15   20   25   30   35   40   45   50   ....

15.   Misuse of equipment/drugs/X-ray films/Reagents etc. is prevalent in Govt. health delivery system.

    0   10   15   20   25   30   35   40   45   50   ....

RAW SCORE   (Please total your response i.e. total 1 to 15).

EFFECTIVE SCORE   (Divided the raw score for each item by 10 and record here)

This represents the "temperature" of the organization

5.2(1)(B) Survey Of Beneficiaries Outside The Ambit Sashastra Seema Bal :

i Methodology:

Another survey of beneficiaries having the same questionnaire, as was provided for the SSB personnel was given to 110 people. The response was more or less the same and the conclusions driven were also particularly the same. Through an error margin of five to ten percent related with the performance indicators can always be considered, while formulating a strategic plan.

ii Summary of results:

Medical health care cost to the patients in the govt. health institution has remained the same/been increasing in the last few years.

Scale		No. of Respondents	Percentage
a.	40	50	45%
b.	30	32	30%
c.	35	28	25%

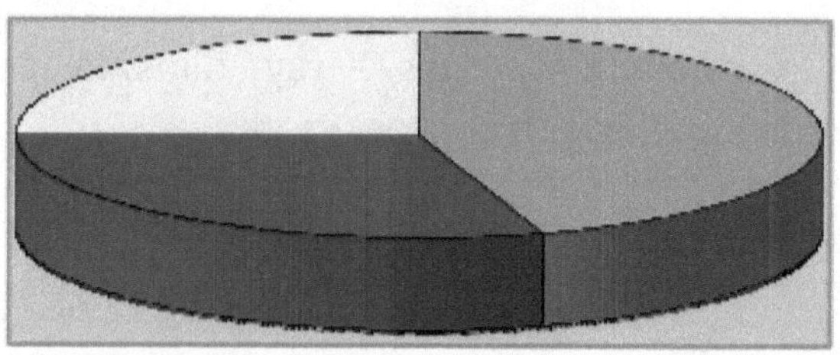

Blue   : 45%

Red   : 30%

Yellow   : 25%

2.   *Government health delivery system provides quality services as per the expectations of patients.*

a.	20	32	30%
b.	25	28	25%
c.	30	50	45%

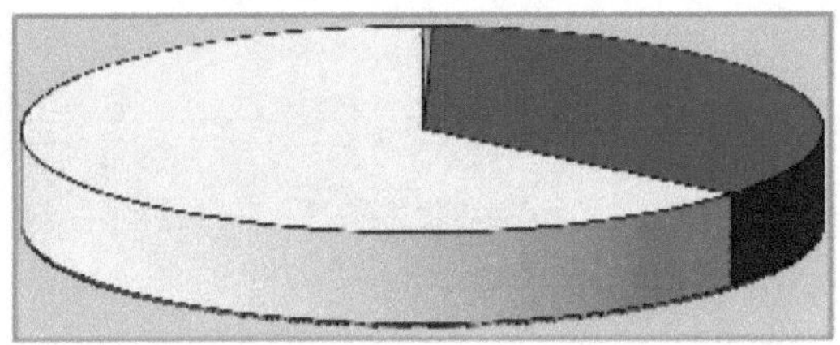

Blue   : 30%

Red   : 25%

Yellow   : 45%

3.   Targets of health programmes are being met.

a.	20	50	46%
b.	40	28	25%
c.	25	32	29%

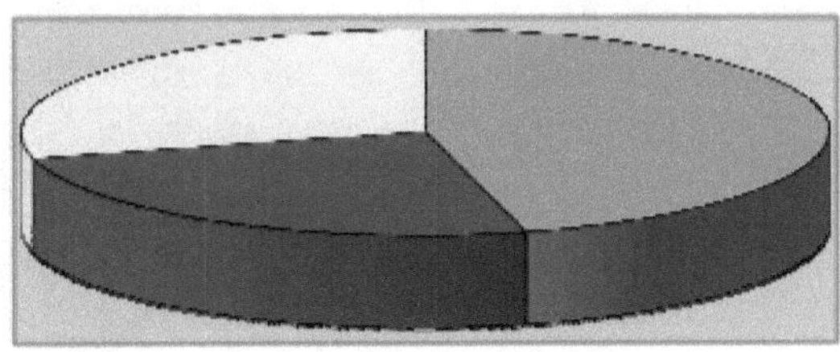

Blue   : 46%

Red   : 25%

Yellow   : 29%

4. Patients/clients complaints regarding poor functioning of govt. hospital/health care.

a.	40	32	30%
b.	45	28	25%
c.	20	50	45%

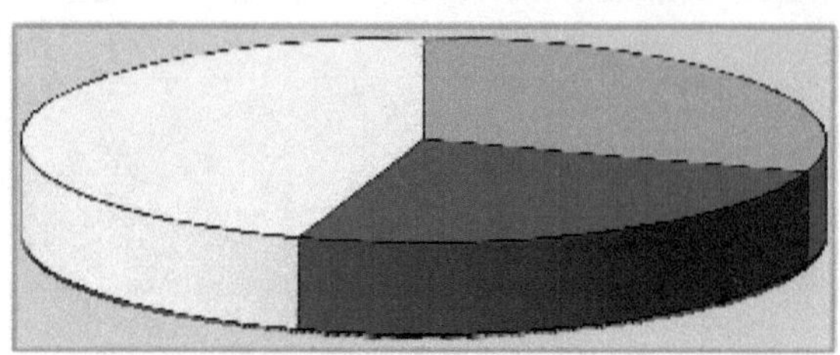

Blue   : 30%

Red   : 25%

Yellow   : 45%

5. Job functions of the team members are not evenly distributed.

a.	40	32	30%
b.	45	28	25%
c.	20	50	45%

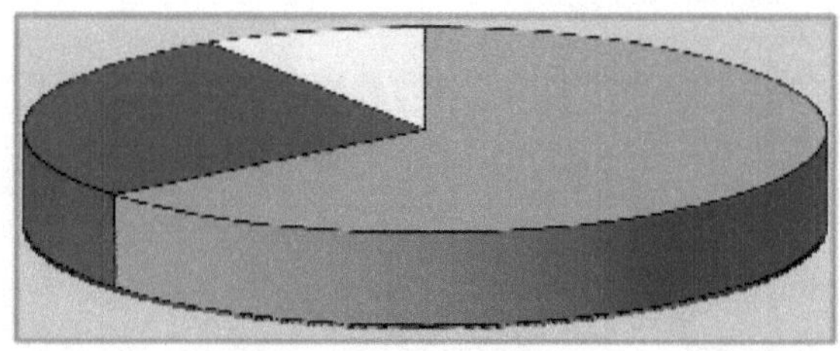

Blue   : 64%

Red   : 27%

Yellow   : 09%

6. Essential drugs in the government hospital/health centers are adequate.

a.	30	35	32%
b.	35	35	32%
c.	40	40	36%

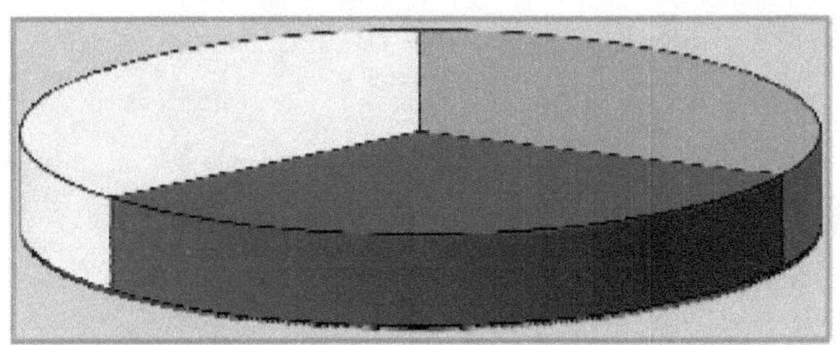

Blue   : 32%

Red   : 32%

Yellow   : 36%

7. Work load on HCW's is more than what can be handled.

a.	30	32	30%
b.	40	28	25%
c.	35	50	45%

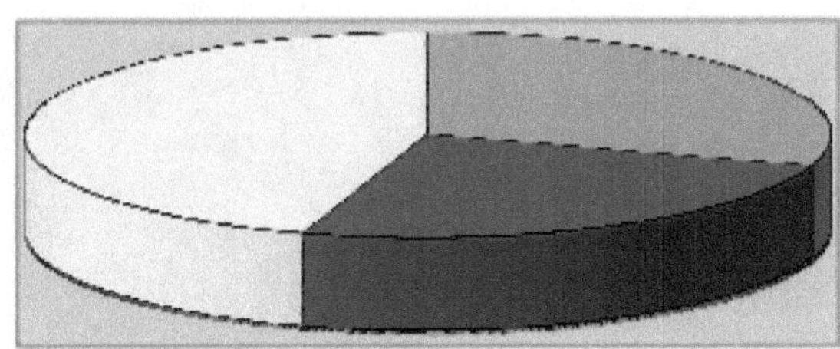

Blue   : 30%

Red   : 25%

Yellow   : 45%

8.   Transfers/posting are frequent and not based on any rationale.

a.	20	32	29%
b.	35	28	26%
c.	40	50	45%

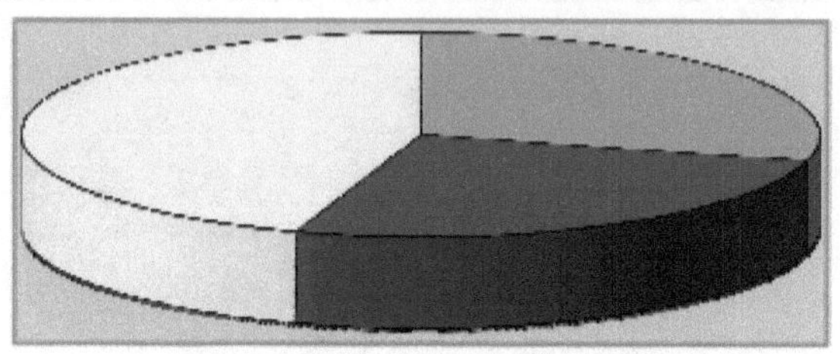

Blue   : 29%

Red   : 26%

Yellow   : 45%

9.   Absentism is a common feature in the govt. health care delivery system.

a.	30	70	63%
b.	25	30	28%
c.	35	10	09%

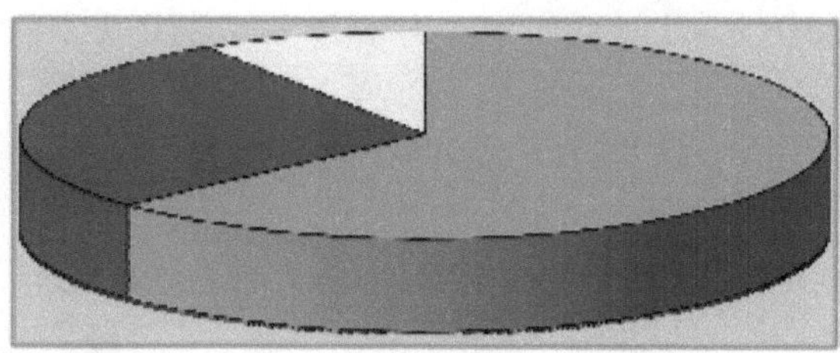

Blue   : 63%

Red   : 28%

Yellow   : 09%

10. Morale of HCW's is low, as compared to other govt. employees.

a.	25	70	64%
b.	30	30	27%
c.	35	10	09%

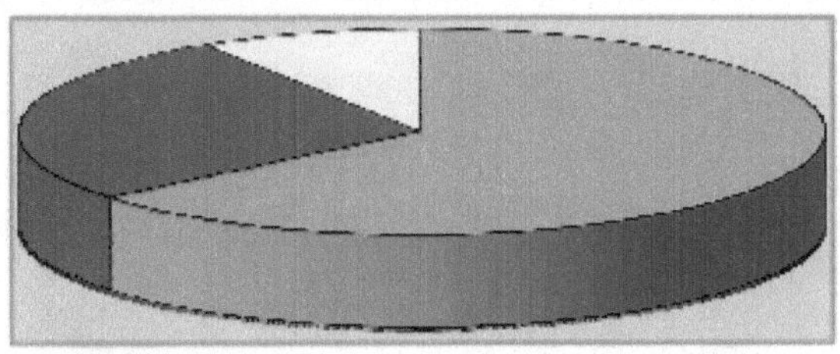

Blue : 64%

Red : 27%

Yellow : 09%

12. Inter –personnel conflicts are common within the health team.

a.	25	32	30%
b.	30	28	25%
c.	35	50	45%

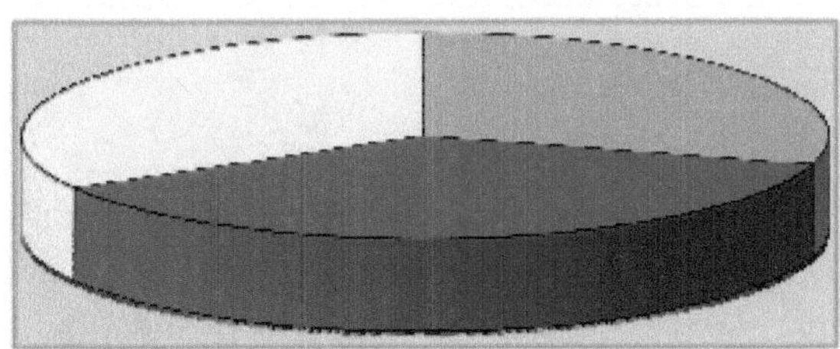

Blue : 30%

Red : 25%

Yellow : 45%

13. Non-compliance with the superior's orders and service rules is common among HCW's.

a.	25	50	45%
b.	35	28	25%
c.	45	32	30%

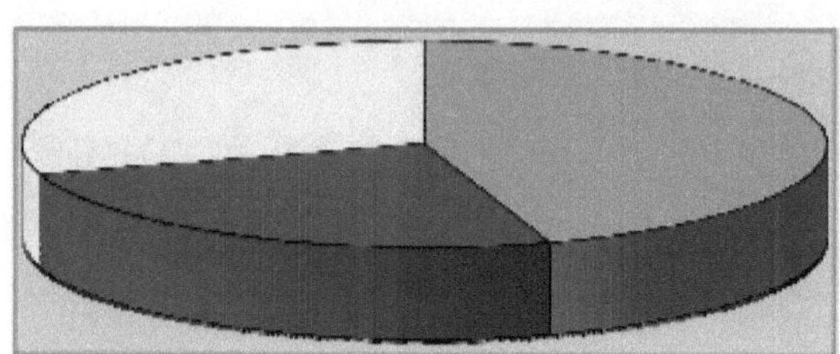

Blue : 45%

Red : 25%

Yellow : 30%

14. Co-operation and co-ordination within the health team is low.

a.	25	32	30%
b.	35	28	25%
c.	45	50	45%

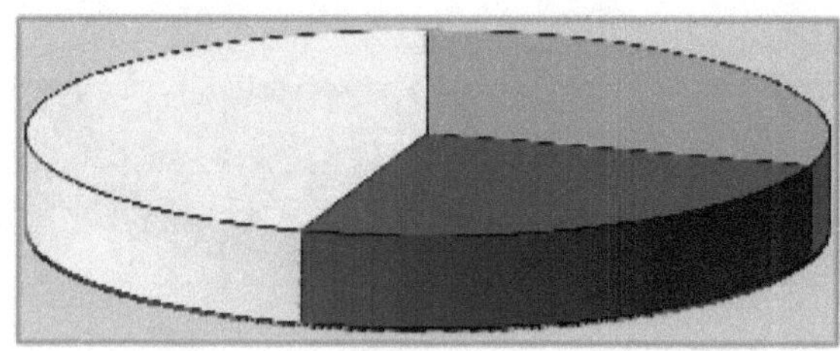

Blue : 30%

Red : 25%

Yellow : 45%

15. Most of non functional equipments in government health institutions require minor repairs.

a.	20	70	63%
b.	35	30	28%
c.	40	10	09%

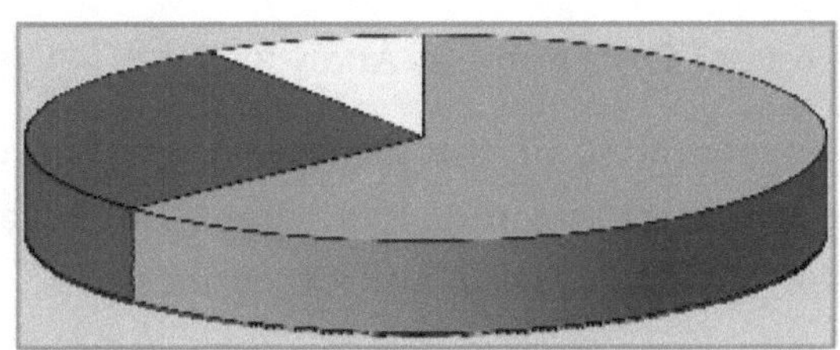

Blue   : 63%

Red   : 28%

Yellow : 09%

16. Misuse of equipments/drugs/S-ray films/ reagents etc is quite common.

a.	25	32	30%
b.	30	28	25%
c.	40	50	45%

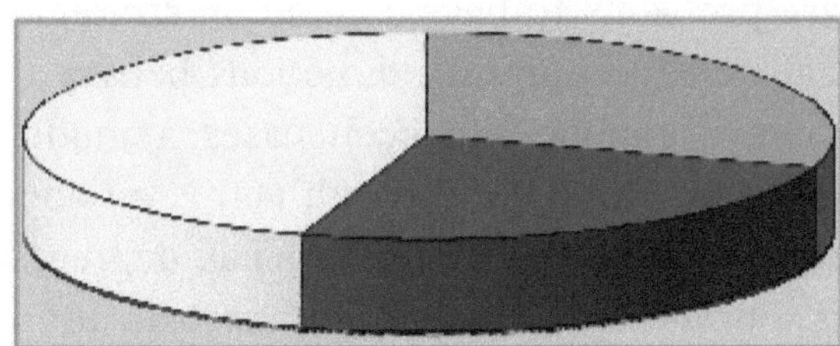

Blue   : 30%

Red   : 25%

Yellow : 45%

5.3 SITUATIONAL ANALYSIS

The analytical process for any strategy formulation is accomplished through these separate methods:

5.3.1 **The External Environment Analysis.**

5.3 .1.1 **The Existing Health Care Systems.**

5.3 .2 **The Internal Environment Analysis.**

5.3. 3 **The Development of the Organization: The development of the organization depends upon the development of–Purpose, Vision, Mission and Objectives.**

5.3.4 **A Gap Analysis: A Gap analysis is done in the form of a SWOT analysis of the SSBHS.**

5.3.5 **Complete Action Plans: It is carried out by developing a Strategic Alternative and strategic Choice.**

5.3.6 **Implementation of the Action Plan: It is the development of the Frontier Level Strategic Plan.** Since, all these three processes (42) are separate entities in themselves, but they generally overlap each other, as such they are basically interacting and influencing each other. To have a perfect fit amongst these three, they are generally dealt with together.

Often there are problems to have a common strategy (43) because of the push and pulls in contrary directions between the external and internal environment. In such cases a muddling through approach is helpful. Muddling through (44) is an approach where the organization moves step by step in small degrees in a forward direction. It is a process of successive approximations towards a desired objective in which what is desired itself continues to change under reconsideration.

5.3 .1 THE EXTERNAL ENVIRONMENT ANALYSIS

A host of influences are involved directly or indirectly in the health care delivery system. Through the decades, the influences that were paramount earlier have changed drastically in the present scenario (45).

A few decades earlier saw physicians, infrastructure, facilities and patients coming under the same roof and working for the betterment of services rendered to the people at large with players like the government departments and business houses staying away from the system, but now the situation has changed so much that private sector business has a hand in the health care delivery system in congruence with the government sector.

The dual relationship that exists between SSB and bordering states on the Indo-Nepal Border is what is important in the present context. What short of external environment exists and how it can be best judged to meet the expectations of the people is what is to be gauged through this study.

THE EXTERNAL ENVIRONMENT ANALYSIS includes

5.3 .1.1 The General Environment around SSBHS.

5.3 .1.2 The Health Care Environment around SSBHS.

5.3 .1.1 THE GENERAL ENVIRONMENT AROUND SSBHS:

Under the following heads the General Environment around SSBHS is discussed.

- a) Government Institutions.
- b) Business Organizations.
- c) Educational Institutes.
- d) Religious Institutions.

e)   Research Organizations and Foundations.

f)   Individuals and Consumers.

a)   **Government Institutions:**

A lot of government institutions are functioning in the states bordering Indo-Nepal both of

The Centre, and

The State.

i   **The Central Govt. Institutions:**

1.   Indian Railway Constructions Ltd. (IRCon).

2.   State Bank of India & others.

3.   Income Tax Department (Ministry of Finance).

4.   Passport Office (Ministry of External Affairs).

5.   Central Reserve Police Force (CRPF) & others.

ii   **The State Govt.Institutions:**

6.   Sikkim Nationalized Transport Corporation (SNTC)

1.   North Bengal State Transport Corporation (NBSTC).

2.   Bihar State Road Transport Corporation (BSRTC).

3.   Sudha Dairy Products.

4.   Himul Dairy Products.

b)   **Business Organizations:**

1.   Sunflower Mall.

2.   Vishal Mega mart.

3.   Mayurya Lok Plaza.

4.   Big Bazaar.

5.   Bata India Limited.

6.   Cosmos mall.

c)   **Educational Institutions**:

     1.   North Bengal University.

     2.   Computer centers.

     3.   Agriculture University.

     4.   Science Colleges (e.g. Patna Science. College)

     5.   Patna University.

d)   **Religious Institutes**:

     1.   ISKCon-Siliguri.

     2.   Patna Sahib-Patna.

e)   **Research Organizations & Foundations-**

     1.   Mahavir Cancer Sansthan & Research Centre.

     2.   Indian Council of Arts & Science.

17.   **(i) Individuals (A select few)**:

     a)   Mr.B.Bhattacharjee (CM-W.B).

     b)   Mr.Nitish Kumar (CM-Bihar).

     c)   Mr. D.Tandon (IG-FTR-SSB-PAT).

     d)   Dr.B.B.Sinha (Director-IRCS).

(ii) Consumers (A select few):

     a)   Common Man.

     b)   Tourists.

     c)   Govt. Departments.

     d)   Private Companies.

5.3 .1.2 THE HEALTH CARE ENVIRONMENT AROUND SSBHS: A discussion will be made about the primary health centre, how it is functioning around, what are the national norms and what are the State protocols. Besides, a short review of the health workers too will be taken up.

Further, these features will be classified under the following heads –

a) ***Organizations that plan and regulate primary and secondary providers.***

b) ***Organizations that provide health services (Primary providers).***

c) ***Organization that provide resources for the health care system (Secondary providers).***

d) ***Organizations that represent the primary and secondary providers.***

e) ***Individuals involved in health care and patients (Consumers of health care services).***

a) ***Organizations that plan and regulate primary and secondary providers***:

State Government regulating agencies:

a) Directorate of health services: Sikkim.W.Bengal, Bihar State.

b) Sikkim, W. Bengal, Bihar State health financing services.

Central Govt. regulating agencies:

a) Director General Health services (MH&FW).

b) Health and Family Planning Department.

c) Public Health Department.

Voluntary regulating groups.

a) The Tata group for social upliftment.

b) The Modis, Escorts groups for ambulatory and rehabilitation services.

c) The Lions International group.

b) ***Primary providers (Organizations that provide health services):***

a) **Hospital**

Govt.

1. The SMC and Hospital.

2. The NBMC & Hospital.

3. The PMC & Hospital.

4. The SKMC & Hospital.

5. The NMC& Hospital.

6. Psychiatry Hospital.

7. Dental Hospital.

8. SSB Hospital.

Investor owned –

1. Suraksha Medical centre.

2. North Bengal Clinic.

3. Magadh Hospital.

4. Dr.Ruben Memorial Hospital.

b) **State Public Health Department.**

c) **Long term care facilities –**

1. Ambulatory services e.g., PMCH

2. Rehabilitation services e.g. Army Hospital, CRPF Hospital, BSF Hospital.

d) Physicians clinics.

e) Home health care – Army, CRPF, BSF.

f) Health Management Organizations (HMO) – Nil.

c) *Secondary providers (Organization that provide resources):*

1. **Educational institutions:**

  i. Medical schools

  ii. NMCH

  iii. PMCH

  iv. NBMCH

  v. School of Nursing

  vi. Health Administration Programs.

2. **Organization that pay for care:**

  i. Government

  ii. Insurance Cos – Mediclaim (By New India Assurance)

  iii. Businesses (e.g. Tata)

  iv. Social organizations (e.g.-Indian Red Cross Society and Rotary Clubs etc.)

3. **Pharmacy and Medical supply:**

  i. Drug distribution (e.g.-Slg Lab Agency)

  ii. Drug and Research companies –

    – Glaxo Company.

    – Torrent Pharmacy.

    – Pfizer.

    – Merck.

4. **Medical Products companies**:

    i.   Bausch and Lomb.

    ii.   Johnson and Johnson.

d) *Organization that represent primary and secondary providers*:

    a)   Indian Medical Association (IMA)

    b)   State Medical Association (GMC & H Association)

    c)   National Medical Organization (NMO)

    d)   Professional Associations (E.g. Pharmaceutical Manf. Association)

e) *Individuals involved in health care and patients (Consumers of health care services)*:

    a)   Physicians

    b)   Nurses

    c)   Pseudo Physicians

    d)   Non-professional physicians

5.3 .1.1 THE EXISTING HEALTH CARE SYSTEMS

i   INTRODUCTORY:

Without going through the existing Health Care systems analysis, the External Environment Analysis does not come to a full stop, as such a short discussion is of paramount importance.

ii   HEALTH CARE SYSTEMS:

OBJECTIVE (*Goal*) : To deliver the "Health Care Services".

CONSTITUTES   : The management sector and involves organizational matters.

OPERATES : In the Socioeconomic & Political framework of the country.

CONSTITUENTS : Known as Sectors/Agencies-5 in number.

    a. Public Sector.

    b. Private Sector.

    c. Indigenous Systems of Medicine.

    d. Voluntary Health Agencies.

    e. National Health Programme.

A. Primary Health Care

    a) Private Hospital

    b) Ayurveda & Siddha

    c) Homeopathy

        – Pr. Health Centers, Poly clinics, Nursing Homes

        – Sub -Centers, Dispensaries.

B. Hospitals/Health Centers

    a) General Practitioners & Clinics.

    b) Comm. Health Centers.

    c) Rural Hospitals.

    d) Distt. Hospitals/Health Centre.

    e) Specialist Hospitals.

    f) Teaching Hospitals.

C. Health Insurance Schemes

    a) ESI

    b) CGHS

D.   Other Agencies

      a)   Defence Services.

      b)   Railways.

*****

[A]   PRIMARY HEALTH CARE:

INTRODUCTORY:

1977   -   GOI launched a "Rural Health Scheme"

      "Placing People's Health in People's hands" (46).

3 tier system -   Based on recommendations of Shrivastava committee in 1975. 1978

      -   Alma Ata- Acceptable level of Health for all by the year 2000 (47).

1983   -   National Health Policy.

      Set to achieve specific goals.

Village Level:

The PH care follows: Universal coverage

Equitable distribution of health resources. For this following schemes are in operation:

Village Health Guides Scheme. Training of local dais.

ICDS scheme.

(1.a.)   Village Health Guides:

Non govt. functionary. Aptitude for social service.

Introduced on 2nd October, 1977.

Launched in all states except Kerala, Karnataka, T.N, A.P. and J & K (In T.N. they have Mini Health centers).

In J & K they have a sub centre – A.D. i.e., Allopathic Dispensary which refer to PHC. Now VHGs are mostly women (In 1986 of GOI replaced guides to W H guides).

Chosen from the community in which they work. 1st link between individual and the health system. Selection Procedure:

- Residents (Permanent) of local area who are women.

- Should be able to read and write minimal education up to 9th standard. Acceptable to all sections of the community.

- Able to spare 2 to 3 hours every day for community Health work.

Post Selection Training:

- 200 hrs spread over a period of 3 months.

- Stipend of Rs. 200 per month.

Post Training:

Receive a working manual and kit of simple medicine of modern and traditional systems.

Duties:

- Simple Medical Ailments.

- Activities in first aid.

- MCH and Family Planning

- Health Education and Sanitation.

N.B.:

1. The manual/ guide book gives detailed information about medical care of common illness when they can start themselves, when they have to refer to the nearest Health Centre.

2. They are free to attend and do community work in their spare time of about 2 to 3 hrs. daily for which they are paid an honorarium of Rs. 50/- PM and drugs worth Rs. 600/- PM.

3. No training by the Govt. for the next 3 years because of cost involvement.

4. 3.24 lacs VHGs in the country.

[1.b.]   *Local Dais:*

A lot of prenatal care during prenatal period for women is available only through Local Dais.

The training programme under RHS (Rural Health Scheme) is to train all categories of local dais (Also called as Traditional Birth Attendants) to enhance their know how about MCH, Sterilization & basic Obstetric skills.

The Duration   :   30 Working days

The Stipend   :   Rs. 300/-

Training Centre   :   PHC/ Sub centre or MCH Centre.

For 2 days in a week.

Rest 4 days to accompany FHW (Female Health Worker).

Supervision of :

FHW

ANM

HA (F)

Strict asepsis to be maintained during delivery.

Total No. of Dais trained from the year 1974 to Sept. 1993: 609750.

(1.c)   Anganwadi Worker:

The literal meaning of Angan means courtyard.

Under ICDS Programme (Integrated Child Development Services) Scheme there is an anganwadi worker for a population of 1000. About 100 workers in each ICDS project.

Present Strength   :   1600

Selection   :   From the community where she stays.

Training   :   4 months upon

Various aspects of

Health Nutrition &

Child development.

Honorarium   :   Part time worker, therefore paid Rs. 200-250/- per Month.

Training includes:

Health Check-up. Immunization.

Supplementary Nutrition. Health Education.

Non formal Pre-school Education, and Referral Services.

Beneficiaries   :

Nursing Mothers.

Other Women (15–45 years). Children (< 6 years).

N.B.:

The village Health Guides and The Anganwadi Workers are the communities' primary link with the Health Services and all other services for young children.

PRIMARY HEALTH CENTRE LEVEL:

Bhore Committee:

1946   -   Bhore Committee – Concept of Primary Health Centre as a basic Health Unit (48).

For integrated, curative and preventive health care for the rural population.

Population: 10,000,-20,000

* 6 Nos.

* 6 Public health nurses

* Other supporting staff.

Couldn't be implement fully even after 40 years.

PHC & Sub centers have visualized them as proper infrastructure to provided health services to the rural population.

Growth of PHC since 1st five year plan – 725.

To 5th five year plan – 5484.

Each PHC has a population of 100,000 or more spread over some 100 villages in each community block. PHC criticized – were not able to provide adequate health coverage. The cause being-

Poorly staffed. Less equipped.

They had to cover a large population (6 or 7 lakhs).

B.   Mudaliar Committee:

1962   - Mudaliar Committee – Regarding strengthening the existing PHC and scaling of population to 40,000.

C.   Alma – Ata Conference:

1978   –   Health for all by 2000 A.D.

             National Health Plan:

1983   –   Reorganization of PHC on the basis of one PHC 20,000 Rural Population in plains 10,000 population in hilly, tribal and backward areas.

PHCs till 1993-21024 against total reorganization of 23,000 by 1990.

Functions:

- Medical care

- MCH including Family Planning.

- Safe Water Supply and Basic Sanitation.

- Prevention and control of locally Endemic Diseases. Collection and Reporting of vital Statistics.

- Education about Health.

- National Health Programme as relevant. Referral Services.

- Training of Health Guides, Health Workers, Local Dais and Health Assistants.

- Basic Services.

SUB-CENTRE LEVEL:

It is the outermost post of the existing health delivery system in the rural areas.

Establishment   :   One for 5000 Population – In general.

                         One for 3000 Population – In hilly, tribal and backward areas.

No. of Sub centers   :   131470

Total Requirement: 1.38 lakhs.

Manpower   : 1.1M- MPHW.

         2.1F - MPHW.

Functions   : Limited to-

         MCH Care.

         Family Planning.

         Immunization.

What Else?

May lead to greater acceptance and easy detection of complication in pregnancy. Supervision by both M & F workers (Health).

Revised norms suggests that one female HA will supervise the work of 6 female HW Job Done:

In accordance with published manuals of the Rural Health Division of the Ministry of H & FW. STAFFING PATTERN

A.	STAFF FOR SUB CENTRE:	NO. OF POSTS.	
1.	Health Worker (Female)/ANM	–	1
2.	Health Worker (Male)	–	1
3.	Voluntary Worker (Paid @ Rs. 50/- PM as honorarium)	–	1
B.	STAFF FOR NEW PRIMARY HEALTH CENTRE:		
1.	Medical Officer	–	1
2.	Pharmacist	–	1
3.	Nurse Mid wife (Staff Nurse)	–	1
4.	Health Worker (Female)/ANM	–	1
5.	Health Educator	–	1
6.	Health Assistant (Male)	–	1
7.	Health Assistant (Female) / LHV	–	1

8.	U.D.C.	-	1
9.	L.D.C.	-	1
10.	Lab Technician	-	1
11.	Driver (Subject to availability of vehicle)	-	1
12.	Class IV	-	4

			15

For every 30,000 population in plain area and 20,000 population in tribal and hilly areas.

C.	STAFF FOR COMMUNITY HEALTH CENTRE:		
1.	Medical Officer	-	4

[Either qualified or specially trained to work as Surgeon, Obstetrician, Physician and Pediatrician. One of the existing Medical Officers similarly should be either qualified or specially trained in Public Health]

2.	Nurse Mid-wives	-	7
3.	Dresser	-	1
4.	Pharmacist/Compounder	-	1
5.	Lab Technician	-	1
6.	Radiographer	-	1
7.	Ward boys	-	2
8.	Dhobi	-	1
9.	Sweepers	-	3
10.	Mali	-	1
11.	Chowkidar	-	1
12.	Aya	-	1
13.	Peon	-	1

		Total:	25

D.   NATIONAL NORMS:

1.	At least one trained Dai	–	for each village.
2.	One trained village Health Guide	–	for each village/1000 population.
3.	One Sub Centre	–	for every 5000 population in plain area and for 3000 population in tribal and hilly areas.
4.	One Primary Health Centre (PHC)	–	for every 30,000 population in plain area and 20,000 populations in hilly and tribal areas.
5.	One Community Health Centre (CHC)	–	for every 80,000 to 1.20 lakh population serving as a referral institution for four Primary Health
	Centers.		
6.	Sub Centers covered by a PHC	–	6 Sub Centers.
7.	PHCs covered by a CHC	–	4 PHCs.
8.	Population covered by a health Worker	–	5000 in plain (Male & Female) area.
		–	3000 in tribal and hilly areas.
9.	Population covered by a Health Asstt.	–	30,000 in plain (Male & Female) area.
		–	20,000 in tribal and hilly areas.
10.	One Health Asstt. (Male & Female)	–	6 health workers (Male/Female).
	Provides supportive supervision to 6 Health workers (Male/Female).		

5.3.2 The Internal Environment Analysis.

INTRODUCTION:

Henri Fayol, a French mining engineer, while writing during the beginning of 20th century stated the following:

"To manage is to forecast and plan to organize, to command, to coordinate, and to control".

Put simply, managing is about assessing probable future scenarios, deciding how best to respond to them, bringing together the resources needed for that response, and deploying them as effectively as possible. Until relatively recently, most management research was concerned with industrial production, for which outputs could be measured relatively easily.

Relatively less attention was given to management of service industries in general and health care services in particular. As Shortell and Kaluzny (1983) noted, *health care services are different from many other organizations. Of course, many of the specificities are differences of degree, with health services sharing many features with other service organizations. Yet important differences exist.*

According to Chester Barnard –

"Unless strategic managers possess a commitment to the organization's purpose and understand the capabilities of the organization, the environment has no meaning....."

– FUNCTIONS OF THE EXECUTIVE.

A *"Distinctive Competence"* is a must if any organization is to survive. SSB *has the unique property of doing things when others are hard* (49) *pressed or least prepared to carry out any given task. Strategy formulation is most of the time nothing but a search for distinctive competence and converting these competencies into unique advantages.*

Services have been developed achieving an important competitive advantage. The study of the internal strengths and weaknesses of SSB can lead to a greater role for professional management in the public sector. Finally, this evaluation of strengths and weakness will lay the foundation for strategic effectiveness of the department.

To understand the SSB culture, the health care systems customary way of thinking must be learnt and subscribed to, by the new members of the staff if they are to be satisfied and productive in their jobs.

Five important subsystems should be considered and detailed study done to assess the strengths and weaknesses of the organization.

What are these five major functional subsystems that should be considered in detail? They are –

1.	Clinical,

2.	Administrative Services,

3.	Marketing,

4.	Finance &

5.	General Management.

The assessment of all these five major functional subsystems should be carried out independently to have their strengths and weaknesses demarcated so as to have a better knowledge for the strategic plan implementation in future.

1.	CLINICAL:

ASSESSING CLINICAL STRENGTHS AND WEAKNESSES:

A.	OPERATIONS STAFF:

[i]	RECOGNISED QUALIFICATIONS:

PHYSICIANS : Few specialists.

NURSES : Nil.

TECHNICIANS: Only few in number.

[i-a]	Documentation & verification is proper.

[I-b]	Excess staff but most specialities lacking.

[i-c]	MORALE: Satisfactory.

[i-d]	INCENTIVES: Provided to the staff.

[ii]   SUFFICIENT NO. OF QUALIFIED
          STAFF (CLINICAL): PHYSICIANS: Needs
          improvement (Because of lack of staff).

[ii-a]   Clinicians not present in adequate number at
          all times.

[ii-b]   Patients in less safer environment due to less
          qualified clinicians.

[ii-c]   Doctors as Clinical Managers-very less.

[ii-d]   Para Medical staff not allowed to judge
          professional matters related to patient care.

[iii]   SUFFICIENT NO. OF QUALIFIED
          TECHNICIANS: TECHNICIANS: Quite a few
          vacancies.

[iii-a]   Technicians meet State licensure /
          registration/ professional certification
          requirements.

[Iii-b]   Technical upgradation is a continuous
          process.

[iii-c]   In-service training opportunities available.

B.   INFORMATION AND INTELLIGENCE:

[i]   Clinical staff has inadequate information
          support system.

[i-a]   Lack of willpower to increase knowledge.

[i-b]   Internal information processing capability is
          inadequate.

[i-c]   Inadequate point record system.

[ii] Satisfactory administrative information systems to process both urgent and routine information.

[ii-a] Occasionally decision making not timely.

[ii-b] Inter communication between physician and other clinical personnel lacking.

[ii-c] Communications not properly documented for allowing professional examination and quality control.

[iii] Procedural lapses in clinical areas inside the SSB arena.

[iii-a] Inadequate links with - State Public Health Department.

         - Centre for disease control.

[iii-b] Competitive rates-information is satisfactory.

C. TECHNICAL CAPABILITIES:

[i] The latest technologies are provided only at a few centers. High quality treatment is provided –as such-only to a few patients.

[i-a] Due to lack of technology or outdated technology staff have a tendency to resign sometimes.

[i-b] Expand and update technology.

[i-c] Radical change lacking in diagnosis & treatment of patients.

[ii] Adequate facilities lacking for comfortable patient care.

[ii-a]   Not dedicated to single purpose use.

[ii-b]   Not dedicated to multi purpose use of facilities.

[ii-c]   Inadequate means of monitoring and evaluating care of patients.

[ii-d]   Protection from toxic elements occasionally provided to the staff.

D.   SYNERGY:

[i]   Para medical staff generally don't understand the value of high quality patient care.

[i-a]   Few organized efforts to reinforce the importance of the highest standards of professional performance.

[i-b]   Regular Medical Education lacking in different specialities.

2.   ADMINISTRATIVE SERVICES:

ASSESSING ADMINISTRATIVE SERVICES STRENGTH AND WEAKNESSES:

A.   ADMINISTRATIVE STAFF:

[i]   Qualified or not:

Administrative Staff   :   Yes.

Managerial Staff   :   Yes

Clerical Support Staff   :   Yes

Data Processing Staff   :   Yes.

[i-a]   Verification, Documentation and training of staff carried out.

[i-b]   Administrative staffs mostly present. Excess staff almost nil.

[i-c]   Good performance on the job front.

[i-d]   Incentive linked performance.

[ii]   Inadequate support staff.

[ii-a]   No provisions for unionization of cadres.

[ii-b]   Competitive wages & benefits for the employees.

[iii]   Properly trained managers.

[iv]   Effective managerial succession plan.

[v]   Proper recruitment in place except in a few cases.

[v-a]   Effective in-service training and development program me for employees at all levels.

[v-b]   Valuable career planning services offered to the staff.

B.   INFORMATION AND INTELLIGENCE:

[i]   Satisfactory information support system present.

[i-a]   Not subscribed to assess data base of high quality health services.

[i-b]   Internal information processing capabilities on the lower side.

[ii]   Inventory control and purchase system is satisfactory. [ii-a] Sufficient information processing capabilities present. [ii-b] Information is effective down the line.

[iii]   Wages and benefit system integrated and accessible to all staff.

[iv]   Clinical intelligence system operates satisfactorily for the purpose of decision making.

[iv-a]   Provision for incentives present.

[iv]   In- house library archives mostly shabbily kept.

[iv-c]   Actions of personnel properly documented and archived.

C.   TECHNICAL CAPABILITIES:

[i]   Insufficient high quality and timely health services present.

[i-a]   Improperly located physical facilities.

[i-b]   Landlocked department.

[i-c]   Unskilled staff in a large number who are not capable to maintain the facilities.

[i-d]   Appropriate parking and unloading facilities present.

[ii]   The administrative support staff doesn't possess the latest technologies.

[ii-a]   Administrative staff not willing to join.

[ii-b]   Updating of documents not up to the mark.

[iii-a]   Automation required for technical and economic reasons.

[iii-b]   OPD be turned into a multiple usage complex.

[iv]   Quality control not up to the mark for the assessment of a persons work.

[iv-a]   Legal council capabilities not up to the mark.

D.   SYNERGY:

[i]   Administrative staff generally interact with all staff members.

    [ii]   Administrative staff members generally satisfy other members of other departments.

3.   ASSESSMENT OF FINANCIAL STRENGTHS AND WEAKNESSES:

A.   FINANCIAL STAFF:

    [i]   Adequate in terms of qualification and number.

    [ii]   Pay and accounts branch to deal with financial matters.

    [iii]   Appropriate and timely data provided by the accounts branch to the executive for proper decision making.

    [iv]   Financial staff responds to special requests for SSBHS.

B.   INFORMATION/ INTELLIGENCE:

    [i]   Appropriate financial information system present.

    [ii]   Necessary archival capacity present to have a base line financial information.

    [iii]   Appropriate data base also present to enhance financial performance.

    [iv]   Archival storage and data bases present to help take financial decisions.

C.   TECHNICAL ISSUES:

    [i]   Absence of cash crunch.

    [ii]   Satisfactory financial growth rate.

D.   SYNERGY:

    [i]   Synergy between finance personnel and other branches.

    [ii]   Accountants don't stop new ideas to take shape.

4.   ASSESSMENT OF MARKETING (PUBLICITY) DEPARTMENTS STRENGTHS AND WEAKNESSES:

A.   MARKETING STAFF:

[i]   Inadequately trained personnel.

[ii]   No Promotional avenues.

[iii]   Publicity officers report to the higher level administrator.

[iv]   Effective interaction between operations and personnel but ineffective between research and development.

B.   INFORMATION/ INTELLIGENCE:

[i]   Publicity provides valuable information about patients treatment facilities.

[i-a]   Geographical origin of patients known.

[i-b]   Sufficient information about services available present.

[i-c]   Referral patients are sent off and on to our facilities.

[ii]   Inadequate marketing information system.

[ii-a] Best available outside support system almost always available.

[ii-b] Inadequate revenue forecast by the marketing staff.

[iii]   Alternative marketing strategies easily developed because of timely information.

[iii-a] Anticipated actions and reactions developed very fast.

[iii-b]   Marketing systems keep people informed about our reputation in the relevant market area (very good in many areas).

C.   TECHNICAL CAPABILITIES:

   [i]   Attainable market goals.

   [ii]   Regular market evaluation.

   [iii]   Effective allocation of marketing resources.

   [iv]   Appropriate marketing mix (Medical, Veterinary and Publicity go hand in glove).

   [v]   Inadequate mechanism to generate and screen new service ideas.

   [vi]   No research and development.

   [vii]   Periodic review does happen regularly.

   [viii]   Services to reach the masses through different source of broadcast.

   [ix]   Promotion of staff at regular intervals needed.

D.   SYNERGY:

   [i]   Effective synergy exists between publicity department and other department of SSB.

   [ii]   Publicity is providing all possible help to market services to new groups of patients and clients.

5.   ASSESSING GENERAL MANGEMENT STRENGTHS AND WEAKNESSES:

A.   MANAGEMENT STAFF:

   [i]   Managers are committed to long term planning process.

[i-a]   Goal setting to be practiced.

[I-b]   Effective communication through out the organization.

[i-c]   Mix between thinking strategically and continuous firefighting required.

[ii]   Use effectively the support staff.

[iii]   Leadership concepts of Managers inadequate besides them being ineffective motivators.

[iv]   Effective budgeting system present.

[v]   Resource allocation based on goal attainment.

B.   INFORMATION/ INTELLIGENCE:

[i]   Up and down flow of information favoured.

[i-b]   Innovative behavior encouraged.

[ii]   Managers not well versed with recent advances in their profession.

[ii-a]   Few managers recognized for their leadership qualities and applauded for the same.

C.   TECHNICAL ISSUES:

[i]   Adequate reward system exists.

[i-a]   The basis of reward may be performance or loyalty.

[i-b]   Performance evaluation is a mix between performance and loyalty.

[ii]   Carefully designed and structured organization.

[ii-a]   Job description however, is not well covered.

[iii]   Sufficient knowledge of organizational history.

[iv]   Sense of security – inadequate sense of security and motivation which needs to be looked into.

D.   SYNERGY:

[i]   A proper design and reengineering required so that different functional sub-systems work not as individual units but as a team.

5.3. 3 THE DEVELOPMENT OF THE ORGANIZATION

5.3.3.1 INTRODUCTION:

The development of the organization depends upon-Purpose, Vision, Mission and Objectives. Based on the questionnaire and Situational Analysis a frame for developing the Purpose, Vision, Mission and Objectives have been developed .Inputs were provided by the founding fathers of the department in question which has been liberally used to develop the above factors.

To reach specific outcomes or goals for SSB Health Services, tools like Purpose, Vision, Mission and Strategic Objectives need to be discussed in detail.

Compared to other branches of SSB the Health Services require a major overhaul in the changed scenario on the INB &IBB.

The SSB is governed by CRPF rules and regulations and was formed in the year 1963 to work in an explosive environment after the Chinese aggression in its role of stay back.

At present SSB has been designated as a border guarding force with deployment on the Indo- Nepal border and Indo Bhutan Border, thereby a paradigm shift has occurred from its stay back role of the decade of sixties. The development of a specific purpose, a specific vision, a specific mission and a specific strategic objective is what is aimed presently in this discussion, especially with special emphasis on SSB health services and that too in the changed scenario.

5.3.3.2 THE PURPOSE:

The purpose of the organizations existence can be traced back to the Chinese aggression way back in the decade of sixties. There was a paradigm shift from the existing Panchsheel and *Hindi-Chini Bhai-Bhai* propounded by Pundit Jawaharlal Nehru.

A sudden attack by the Chinese army (63, 64) took away more than twelve thousand square kilometers of India in the Arunachal region-the then North Eastern Frontier Area (NEFA). Tens of thousands of civilians and army personnel were injured/killed in the attack of sudden proportions.

At that particular time the planners of modern India envisaged a role where an organization could work in such drastic conditions for the welfare of the suffering population, the wounded jawans and so on and so forth.

Thus, the purpose of SSB was propounded suggesting a stay back role in conditions of utter adversity. Then in 1963 SSB came in to being. From then to now it has grown leaps and bounds but the basic purpose remains the same-i.e.,-Service, Sacrifice & Brotherhood.

5.3.3.3 THE VISION:

The vision for SSB has been nothing but the founders philosophy which suggests starting an organization which brings home both nursing and hospital care.

This expression of hope has resulted in a modest research, teaching and patient care facility. Though patient care facility is quite good, the teaching and research facility has to mend roads.

The vision envisaged prevention to replace cure. Again this aspect has been in the forefront and somewhat met halfway.

Another aspect of vision for SSB is the role of a catalyst, evaluates and motivates, operating network of information and feedback with other government and private agencies.

To integrate appropriate technology, to support efforts in not for profit health care at all levels especially the bordering villages and hilly terrain.

To integrate education and health care practice for a holistic approach so as to safeguard the trust between health care workers of SSB and the community at large.

To be expert, flexible and mobile in the face of disaster, these three ethos are almost always associated with the vision of SSB functionaries.

To move further with the changing times, but keeping the past influences for stimulating the work culture of the future generations to come.

To develop strategies of human resource development, to enhance communication skills, facilitate job satisfaction for all SSB personnel and allied departments.

To develop a vital role for SSB for achieving health for all in the States where it is situated by adequate medical coverage in association with other departments strategically associated with SSB.

Such effective vision envisaged for SSB was propounded by our late Prime Minister Smt. Indira Gandhi and later Shri. Rajeev Gandhi, another doyen of Indian heritage giving his full support to this visionary aspect for a better future for the Indian people. As such SSB has become a, "a beacon in the midst of chaos" in the present environment.

5.3.3.4 THE MISSION STATEMENT:

The founding fathers of SSB were visionaries. Yet a mission statement had been lacking. A philosophy for SSB was propounded in the form of Service, Sacrifice and Brotherhood. On the basic of these, a well conceived mission has been created, which is more concrete than a vision. It is an attempt to capture the essence of the organizational purpose and give it a concrete shape.

Sometimes, the thinking moves in a haphazard way and people tend to forget the mission statement, but the true keepers of the vision have a role, especially during times of crisis to motivate people which are based on the mission statement.

Some important characteristics that a mission statement should have are as follows:

    i   Broadly defined statements.

    ii   Should be enduring.

    iii   Should underscore the uniqueness of the organization.

    iv   Should be specific as regards to scope of operations in terms of service.

In the light of the above mentioned broad based classification a mission statement for SSB health services is illustrated as follows:

A Mission Statement for SSBHS:

SSBHS, is a central government, not for profit country level centre, whose mission is to – Provide comprehensive health care services to patients appropriate for their special needs.

Provide leadership, experience and expertise as a community and state resource to augment the health and welfare of people living in remote peripheral villages of bordering states.

Provide education and training to health care workers committed for the welfare of such unprivileged people of bordering states.

Understand health problems of the people which geriatric problems and those who are terminally ill. Provided service to the local people, security for ill patients and stopping breach of trust by spreading brotherhood between all and sundry.

Emphasize the health services commitment to team efforts to gain the desired effect amongst the local populace.

Collaborate with community organizations to develop a community base health protection system for vulnerable population especially fire from across the border.

Vulnerable populations are:

i   Villages under direct line of fire.

ii   Inpatient who need day care.

iii Prenatal/post partum/ child care services.

iv   Geriatric population

v   Mentally ill, retarded and chemically dependent individuals.

vi   HIV/AIDS patients & Drug Addicts.

The SSB is committed to the upliftment of the disadvantaged and vulnerable groups of the society, especially those who are living in the far-flung and remote hilly areas of the country, especially in the bordering states.

Finally SSB aims at assisting individuals achieve their highest potential through educational tours and trips and endeavors to promote mental, physical and spiritual well being.

5.3.3.5 THE OBJECTIVES (GOALS):

Based on the exhaustive studies duly carried out as mentioned through chapters 2 to chapter 5 (Direct - Survey of SSB personnel, Survey of External Beneficiaries; Indirect - Published work etc.

and External and Internal Environmental Analysis besides Existing Health Care System Analysis) the strategic goals and objectives for SSBHS have been summarized below. However some Key Performance areas need emphasizing upon. The key performance areas that need emphasis are as follows:Nutrition, Physical fitness, Tobacco, Alcohol and Drugs/HIV/AIDS, Sexual Behavior, Violent and Abusive Behavior, Anemia Correction, Promote Family Planning, Prevent Complications, Help of trained local dais and female health workers, Anti malarials, Tetanus Prophylaxis, Vitamin A Supplementation, Environmental Health, Occupational Safety and Health.

KEY PRIORITY AREAS:

Key priority areas related with Preventive & Management Aspects which are as follows:

HIV/STD infection, Drug Deaddiction, Cancer, Oral hygiene, Mental and behavioral discrepancies, Health education training and preventive services, Surveillance, Caretaker support system. ***Say for example M.M.R. (Maternal Mortality Rate) in 1988 in developing countries was 505 and in India our aim is to lessen it by 2 from 3-4 (in 1988) per thousand live births. As such it has been prioritized as a strategic objective.*** Infant mortality rates are strategically planned to be reduced to less than sixty by the year 2010 A.D. Though these points are only a pointer to why they have been prioritized still they can be considered as exemplary areas but not exhaustive as such. Other indicators can be summed up through Infant Mortality Rate, Health and Fertility Programs by region, Child Death Rates and Child Survival Rates.

Based on the above priority areas and exhaustive studies duly carried out as mention through chapters 2 to chapter 6 (Direct - Survey of SSB personnel, Survey of External Beneficiaries; Indirect - Published work etc. and External and Internal Environmental Analysis besides Existing Health Care System Analysis and Identifying Burning

Issues like Drug Addiction and Obesity etc.) the strategic goals and objectives for SSBHS have been summarized below. These broad goals and objectives represent the mission of the SSBHS encompassing its prime functions.

SSB HS STRATEGIC PLAN – GOALS AND OBJECTIVES – FY 2007-2012

Goal 1 : Quality Health Care and Infrastructure Development: Increase safety & quality, affordability and accessibility of health care, including behavioral health care and long term care.

Objective 1.1 Widen long-term care coverage.

Means of accomplishing the objective: Improving upon record keeping provisions at different points in time & different places in Question.

Objective 1.2 Improve availability and accessibility of health care services.

Means of accomplishing the objective: Increase the number of available access points providing care to vulnerable and special needs population.

Objective 1.3 Improve health care outcome, safety, cost and value through improved infrastructure development.

Means of accomplishing the objective: Expand development of already developed buildings, Labs, Pathology units and Emergency services including Outpatient (OP) and Inpatient (IP) services.

Objective 1.4 Recruit, develop through appropriate treatment protocol and retain a competent health care workforce and Para Medical Staff.

Means of accomplishing the objective: Provide training opportunities and technical assistance besides recruitment of new staff. Recruitment to be carried out in far-flung areas and also where facilities of health care are partially existing or non- existent like Nathula in Sikkim nearing Chinese Border.

Goal 2 : Health Promotion and protection, prevention of disease and Prepare for any contingency/Emergency:

Prevent and control disease, injury, illness and disability across the life span, and protect the SSB Personnel/public (5 Kms from the border) from infectious, occupational, environmental disease and terrorist attacks.

Objective 2.1 Infectious disease spread prevention and effective control of HIV/AIDS through VCCT centers, besides Malaria, Kalazar, Diarrhoea and Dysentry.

Means of accomplishing the objective: Target VCCT resources to infected people with HIV/AIDS directly.

Target PHCs and MI Room resources to individuals suffering from infective disease.

Objective 2.2 Protect the SSB Personnel/ public against injuries and environmental disease/ threats. ***Means of accomplishing the objective:*** Providing maximum resources to personnel/public through the PHC's/MI Room's and Composite Hospitals.

Objective 2.3 Encourage & promote preventive health care including mental health (Psychosomatic disorders), communicable disease and lifelong healthy behavior through Drug Deaddiction camps/ centers.

Means of accomplishing the objective: Increase participation of eligible individuals receiving care through Government of India- Ministry of Health and Family Welfare funded programmes having Preventive and Chronic Disease treatment services (i.e. Immunization, Psychosomatic disorders, Drug Deaddiction Camps etc.)

Objective 2.4 Prepare for and respond to natural and manmade disasters and terrorist attacks/contingency/emergency.

Means of accomplishing the objective: Increased training and preparedness for facing any eventually in case of emergency.

Goal 3 : Service to Mankind through WARB (Welfare and Rehabilitation Board): Promotion of economic and social well-being of SSB personnel, individuals, families & communities.

Objective 3.1 Promote the economic independence and social well-being of SSB personnel, individuals and families on the INB & otherwise.

Means of accomplishing the objective: Utilizing Empanelled hospitals for the well being of patients from SSB and otherwise.

Objective 3.2 Promote safeties and wellbeing of children and youth of SSB & on the INB.

Means of accomplishing the objective: Pulse Polio Immunization Programme to be implemented in toto.

Objective 3.3 Develop strong, healthy, and supportive communities for both SSB personnel & population on the INB through WARB especially for physically handicapped personnel.

Means of accomplishing the objective: WARB facilities to be utilized for rehabilitation of Physically Handicapped Personnel.

Objective 3.4 Analyze strengths, weakness and abilities of SSB personnel as well as vulnerable population on the INB to nullify health disparities.

Means of accomplishing the objective: Train Para Medical Staff and Doctors to be more effective and annul weaknesses if any. Train population on the borders to be abreast of recent advances on the border on health and healthy practices and medical updates.

Goal 4 : Research and development with increasing management practices: Enhance research and development related to health and human services on the INB.

Objective 4.1 Increase the pool of qualified culturally diverse health and Para Medical Staff through

a)   New & wide ranging training programme and

b)   Assured career progression under SSBHS in rural & border areas.

Means of accomplishing the objective: Enhance electronic training programmes for Para Medical Staff and Medical Profession. Monitor and Evaluate electronic resources (e.g. Web sites, list server, data system for Ministry of Health and Family Welfare and SSBHS granters and funded programmes).

Objective 4.2 Increase basic Medical knowledge to improve human health & mass management. *Means of accomplishing the objective:* CME for Medical Professionals both in house and through distant mode through electronics media as well as at Testing Care Centers like Composite Hospitals and Research Centers (IGIMS & NBMCH, PMCH etc.) Complete Management Protocol to be followed through short and long term training programmes.

Objective 4.3 Conduct and oversee applied research to improve health and well-being.

Means of accomplishing the objective : Promote applied research programme by the Medical professionals specially on issues related with Colour Blindness and P.F Malaria, HIV/AIDS infections/ Drug Deaddiction/ Preventive & Social Medicine/Obesity and Hypertension etc.

Objective 4.4 Communicate and transfer research results into clinical, public health and human service practice including achieving excellence in management practices.

Means of accomplishing the objective: The results so achieved be transmitted to group of Para Medical Staff and Medical Professional directly associated with patient care.

Summary:

To attain the strategic objectives envisaged for SSB by the year 2012 in league with other brother departments, it is imperative that the Strategic Objectives be given the top priority amongst other engagements along with the study providing different inferences at different times.

5.3. 4 A Gap Analysis:

A Gap analysis is done in the form of a Strength Weakness, Opportunities & Threats **(SWOT) analysis of the SSBHS.** Typically, this step involves examining the organization through use of a SWOT analysis (strengths, weaknesses, opportunities and threats). Organizational strengths may include longevity, experience of personnel and security of assets. On the other hand, weaknesses can include lack of a change mentality, being asset-rich and cash-poor, and a high employee turnover rate. Opportunities generally take the form of a competitive advantage of some sort such as a one-of-a-kind product, lower manufacturing costs, or breakthrough technology.

Threats are considered when developing strategic plans, though usually not in the same manner that contingency planners view them. While a contingency planner may view a threat as being a natural or technological event, strategic planners may look at threats more in terms of competitors and loss of market share. Other factors can impact an organization and be classified as threats, for example, pending state or federal regulations, zoning laws, economic trends, and so forth.

The Threats, Opportunities, Weakness & Strength Analysis:

STRENGTHS	**WEAKNESSES &PROBLEMS**
CLINICAL:	1. CLINICAL:
* Proper verification & documentation of qualification	*Few Specialists, PMS.
* All Technicians meet State Licensure/Registration /Prof.	* Excess staff at few places (Eg. Certification. Directorate level)
*. Technicians abreast with current/ latest methods.	* Satisfactory Morale.
* In-service training opportunities available.	* Less professional judgment
=> High quality treatment provided	=> Inadequate information for Clinical staff.
* Dedicated to single purpose use of facilities [Eg. Providing advanced training before recruitment of Local population].	* High quality treatment provided, but at a few centers only.
* Dedicated to multipurpose use of facilities [Eg. Some Orators and also trained in in-house training.	* Irregular meeting of different clinical Clinicians are specialists, as well as Journalists as well as good specialties.
* Not all Cl. Staff understand and share common	
=> Casual/annual medical of staff.	Goal of high quality pt. care.

2. ADMINISTRATIVE:

2. ADMINISTRATIVE:

* Well trained, qualified managerial staff.	* No valuable career planning service offered to the employees.
* Effective in-service training & development prog.	* No effort to assess database of high quality health service.
* Competitive wage & benefits compared with Other employees in the area.	* Dilapidated in-house Library.
* Effective inventory control & purchase system.	* Landlocked department.
* Effective & sufficient information processing Capabilities present down the line.	* Less of latest technology.
* Provisions for incentives to managers and present.	* Automation required. Workers

* Excellent synergy between different
sub units.

3. FINANCES	3. FINANCES

* Very good staff, in terms of
qualifications & number.

* Ego-centric attitude of a few
Personnel.

* No payment to external financial
services.

* New ideas occasionally cold
Shouldered.

* Accounting matters provided timely
date for Proper decision making.

* Appropriate financial info. System.

* Necessary archival data base present .

* No cash crunch.

* Satisfactory rate & financial growth

* Synergy between finance & other
departments.

4. MARKETING (PUBLICITY):	4. MARKETING (PUBLICITY):

* Effective interaction between
operations & personnel

* No R & D programme.

* Valuable information about patient
base.

* Inadequate trained personnel.

* Geographical origin of pts. Fully
known.

* Use of best available outside support
system almost always, e.g. Audiovisual
aids.

* Anticipated actions & reaction
developed very fast.

* Marketing systems keep people
informed about our reputation in the
relevant product area (Very good in
many areas)

* Regular marketing evaluation.

* Effective allocation of marketing
resources.

* Appropriate marketing mix between
Medical Veterinary & Publicity.

* Periodic review done.

* Excellent synergy between SSB and other departments.

* All possible help to market services to new groups of Patients & clients.

5. MANAGEMENT:

* Long term planning.

* Effective communication.

* Resource allocation based on goal attainment.

* Mop-down management system.

* Few managers recognized for their leadership qualities.

* Adequate revival system exists.

* Performance evaluation is a mix between performance & loyalty.

* Carefully designed & structured organization.

5. MANAGEMENT:

* A mix reqd. between thinking strategically & Continuous firefighting.

* Ineffective motivators, role models for the Younger generation employees.

* Suggestions by employees rarely considered,

* Proper redesign re-engineering required.

OPPORTUNITIES

1. CLINICAL:

* Recruit Physician Specialists in selected fields.

* Expand home health services.

* Medical/nursing student's services can be improved further.

* Improve Emergency & OPD services.

* Strive to shape public policy to improve health.

THREATS & RISKS

1. CLINICAL:

* Staff resign sometime because of outdated & /insufficient technology.

* Physical facilities inadequate at some places for comfortable patient care.

* Proper expertise lacking for employees in case Of war or nuclear holocaust.

2. ADMINISTRATIVE

* Establish all services depts. To attract tech. qualified Specialists & staff.

* Affiliated with larger hospitals.

2. ADMINISTRATIVE:

* Less attractive to technically qualified staff.

* Usage of existing facilities less.

3. FINANCES:

* Resource allocation from R & D programme.

3. FINANCES:

* Tendency to overspend.

4. MARKETING (PUBLICITY)

* Market holding capacity can be increased. (of valuable info. about patients).

* Other departments refer patients to our Facilities especially during Emergency.

* Best possible support system present almost always (CT Scan, MIR etc.)

* Alternative Marketing Strategies developed before others can have an idea of it.

4. MARKETING (PUBLICITY):

* Promotional avenues not filled in time.

* Inadequate machinery to generate & re run New service ideas.

5. MANAGEMENT:

* Can assist people in taking responsibility about their health.

* Preference for the economically poor and deprived.

* Maximum reimbursement from third party payers.

* Hire & retain qualified employees.

* Increase community & consumer awareness via marketing & Community solutions.

5. MANAGEMENT:

* Inadequate leadership at many levels.

* Existing managers have a tendency to job-hop.

* Job description for managers not pinpointed.

5.3.5   Complete Action Plans:

It is carried out by developing a Strategic Alternative and strategic Choice.

The Strategic Alternative:

(Selected at the SSB Frontier level)

1. **The Alternatives**: The Alternatives available at the three levels are as follows:

    A. **Secretariat (Corporate) Strategies -**

        i. **Growth -**

           Diversification

           Vertical Integration

        ii. **Degeneration -**

           Divestiture

           Liquidation

    B. **Frontier (Divisional) Strategies -**

        i. **Growth -**

           Market Share Building

           Market Share Holding

           Turnaround

        ii. **Degeneration -**

           Market Share Harvesting

           Retrenchment.

    C. **Functional Strategies –**

        i. Marketing

        ii. Finance

        iii. Organization & Staffing.

(ii)   The Selected Frontier (Divisional) Level Alternatives:

The selected Frontier (Divisional) level alternatives are as follows:

Related Diversification.

Vertical Integration.

Market Share Building & Holding.

Related Diversification: No organization can grow by itself hence a bit of diversification in related fields is called for.

A potential for substantial growth, if it exists outside the organization - then it should be utilized for the betterment of the Frontier. If the products and markets are selected carefully, a complimentary relationship can be developed for the mutual benefit of each other. Having a skilled technical staff for intensive care patients can be thought of in terms of product/ service area.

Why Related Diversification will be helpful in the case of SSB Health Services is because of its large reach towards its customers. Working on the INB, going towards each and every far-flung area and interacting with the people can build advantageous positions especially in fields like –

- – In-home Transfusion Therapy.

- – In-home Physical Therapy.

- – Community Health Counseling.

- – Outpatient Investigation Processes (Eg. USG, CT Scan)

- – Hematology/Biochemistry, etc.

- – Outpatient Diagnostic Services (Eg. Cardiovascular Services).

- – Family Planning, Parenting & Immunization Services.

- Occupational Health Services.

- Primary Health Care Group Practice.

***Vertical Integration*:** Vertical Integration Strategy is a decision to grow along the channel of distribution of the core-operations.

It may be of two types:

    i   Towards Suppliers (Upstream) (Backward Integration)

    ii   Towards Patients (Downstream) (Forward Integration)

In case of SSB Health Services, the forward Integration or downstream towards the patients is what the alternative strategy calls for.

Though backward integration is definitely called for, but since the organizational structure is such that a top down management decision is concentrated towards the patients. Hence a forward integration process is called for.

    i   ***Market Share Building & Holding:***

    ii   ***Market Share Building*** is a decision to grow in the present market or to enter new markets with present products or services.

With the number of strengths and opportunities present in the SSB organizations Health Services at the Frontier (Divisional) Level, Market Share Building and Holding can both go hand in glove. Another aspect is being dealt by "Horizontal Integration" which is primarily purchasing direct competitors and is primarily a Market Share Building process. Here the SSB organization can build on professional customers by purchasing or going into a joint venture with say CRPF, BSF etc.

***Market Share Holding*:** Market Share Holding is nothing but Stabilization and Maintenance Strategy. Its basic goal is to maintain services at current levels.

This strategy is appropriate when there are two or three dominant providers in a stable market segment, as is found in the SSB context where the CRPF, BSF the Army and different Health Services are working side by side. By providing service which are cost effective, easily available and sensitive to the sensibilities of the local population, SSB Health Services can hold on to its market share.

An example is providing excellent medical care even during cordon and search, heavy infiltration from across the border. Thus, aspects like Marketing, Publicity, Finances and Organization and Staffing too are maintained together.

In any of these three aspects the help of generic strategies too can be taken which are-

i **Cost Leadership:** Cost leadership is providing best possible facility in the least possible cost. If SSB has to be the cost leader it should try aggressively to -

Construct efficient facilities. Reduce costs.

Control on overheads.

Research & Development to be prioritized.

ii **Differentiation:** What the other departments produce or service and what SSB does is called differentiation.

SSB service should be seen as unique among a group of similar workers.

The ease of access, reporting, convenience etc. are features on which SSB Health Services can work upon to be different from other market players.

iii **Focus:** Focus is a specific, well defined "niche" in the total market that SSB wants to pursue in the present situation providing "Easy *access to emergency medical care for all especially in the remotest part of INB that is not only cost* *effective but well differentiated from other similar service providers – is what is the focus of the SSB Health Services."*

Thus, *The Strategic Choice (Alternatives)*: Market Share Building (For SSB Health Services at Frontier (Division) Level).

***The* SSB FRONTIER *(Divisional)* Positioning Strategy: Cost effective, well differentiated focused.**

"Easy access to emergency medical care for all, especially in the remotest part of Indo-Nepal Border that is not only "cost effective" but "well differentiated "from the other similar service providers is what is the "focus" of the SSB Health Services.

CONCLUSION:

To conclude, Market Share Building, Which is cost effective, well differentiated and focused at the Frontier (Divisional) Level should be the Strategic Alternative & Strategic Choice.

5.3.6. Implementation of the Action Plan:

It is the development of the Frontier Level Strategic Plan.

The Strategic Plan at the Frontier (Divisional) level for SSB Health Services can be traced through the earlier discussions as follows:

1. **THE STRATEGIC CHOICE (ALTERNATIVES):**

    Market share building.

2. **THE SSB FRONTIER(DIVISIONAL) POSITIONING STRATEGY:**

    Cost Effective. Well Differentiated. Focused.

    Easy access to emergency medical care for all especially in the remotest part of Indo Nepal Border, that is not only Cost effective but well differentiated from other similar service providers is what is the focus of the SSB Health Services.

3. **STRATEGIC DECISION AREAS:**

   A. **Mission:**

   " ...The SSB is committed to the upliftment of the disadvantaged and vulnerable groups of the society, especially those who are living in the far-flung and remote hilly areas of the country, especially in the bordering states."

   B. **Customer Mix:**

   Health for all On Indo Nepal Border and adjacent regions especially Emergency Medical Aid, Health and Family Welfare, Geriatric and Pediatrics population care.

   C. **Product Mix:**

   Primary Health Care, excellent emergency treatment under heavy Insurgency & Terrorism, Pediatric, Geriatric, Rehabilitation, Nursing, Surgical, Drug Deaddiction, HIV/AIDS and other related services and disease.

   D. **Service Area:**

   Indo Nepal Border and adjacent areas.

   E. **Goals and objectives:**

   Health for all

   High level of emergency care

   Decrease infant mortality role, prenatal mortality role, crude birth rate, family size.

   Increase immunization coverage. Innovative treatment

   Up gradation of surgical, Geriatric and Pediatric services.

F.   **Competitive Advantage:**

Great image.

High quality service.

Widely recognized staff (especially with the Army, CRPF, BSF). State Health Services.

Grant financial, Publicity and Administrative advantage.

G.   **Outside relationships:**

Excellent relationship with State Health services, Army, CRPF, BSF. MCI recognition.

High commendation from the Ministry of Home Affairs and other international organizations (e.g. WHO)

Conclusion:

The Frontier Level Strategic Plan –as such is based on Market Share Building where the SSBHS is on a solid ground, thereby suitable action can be taken for its further upliftment in the times to come.

Chapter 6
CONCLUSIONS & RECOMMENDATIONS

6.1 MARKET SHARE BUILDING:

VIA: MINOR & MAJOR MEDICAL CIVIC ACTIONS.

6.2 MEDICAL:

*COST CONTROL WITH QUALITY TREATMENT.

*EQUIPMENT MAINTENANCE WITH INFRASTRUCTURE DEVELOPMENT.

*PROVISIONS FOR ESSENTIAL DRUGS.

*AUGMENT EXISTING HOSPITAL FACILITIES, CME (CONT. MEDICAL EDUCATION), TRAINING & PRACTICE SESSIONS (FOR CLINICAL & PM STAFF).

*PROVISIONS FOR POTABLE DRINKING WATER TO ERADICATE GASTRO-ENTERITIS & RELATED DISEASE.

*HEALTH & FAMILY WELFARE PROGRAMME TO BE HANDLED MORE EFFICIENTLY.

6.3 MANAGEMENT & ADMINISTRATIVE:

A.   ASSURED CARRER PROGRESSION.

B.   CO-ORDINATION BETWEEN STAFF OF SSBHS & SHS.

C.   AVOID FREQUENT TRANSFERS/POSTINGS

D.   PROPER JOB DISTRIBUTION.

E.   PROPER SECURITY FOR MEDICAL PERSONNEL. (FROM: SHELLING, CORDON & SEARCH ETC.)

F.   RETRAIN/TRIM PARTIALLY TRAINED/UNSKILLED STAFF.

G.   AUTOMATION/COMPUTERISATION REQUIRED FOR TECHNICAL & ECONOMIC REASONS.

6.4 PUBLICITY (MARKETING):

RESEARCH & DEVELOPMENT.

RETRAIN/TRIM PARTIALLY TRAINED/UNSKILLED STAFF. HEALTH FOR ALL.

The SSB is committed to the upliftment of the disadvantaged and vulnerable groups of the society, especially those who are living in the far-flung and remote hilly areas of the country, especially in the bordering states.

SSB aims at assisting individuals achieve their highest potential through educational tours and trips and endeavors to promote mental, physical and spiritual well-being.

As such some basic themes have surfaced repeatedly during this study, which can be recommended for implementation for the overall benefit & development of SSB Health Services.

First of all, what needs curing is not just too little market or too much market. The expansion of market is among the instruments that can help to promote human capabilities and given the imperative need for rapid elimination of economic deprivation in India, it would be irresponsible to ignore that opportunity.

In this context, the strategic alternative in the form of Market Share Building is very important especially where SSBHS has a strong potential to win over the local populace with its Minor & Major Civic Action (Medical) Programmes.

Coming to the medical part be it clinical or Para clinical utmost emphasis must be given to cost control without sacrificing on quality treatment.

Essential drugs, equipment maintenance and meeting health targets (like Health for all) should be top priority areas.

*A strategy can be developed to augment the existing hospital facilities for in house, on-the-job training and practice sessions, especially in case a strategy is to be followed at the divisional and functional level.

*Provisions for potable drinking water to eradicate Gastro enteritis & related diseases can be given their due.

*Health and Family Welfare Programmes should be handled with more efficiency.

*Control of TB as well as detection of TB between jawans living in hard living conditions leading to over crowding can not be over emphasized. A long term as well as short term / operational objective of treatment and detection by investigation can be considered as an interest for the SSB Para Medical Staff specially the civilian component who have been rendered defunct because of change in the role of SSB once it was deployed on Indo Nepal Border and Indo Bhutan Border.

In the changing scenario the SSB health services especially the Para Medical Staff can also take care of the border population, which is primarily in the area of responsibility of SSB.

A direct surveillance through Para Medical Staff and Doctors can go a long way in establishing control of TBC in and around Indo Nepal Border and eradicating TBC.

*SSB being on the Indo Nepal Border can given a good input to the central Government especially in the DARJEELING district, SILIGURI township & NAXALBARI area which are falling in its working zone. Health services are -as such- required to be augmented and the services of Para Medical Staff trained in such demographic data collection can be utilized for national redressal of leprosy.

*Since, about eighty percent of the deployment of SSB is on the Indo Nepal Border and Indo Bhutan Border which is basically village population and that too with rural background of the border villages – it can be emphasized with specifications that the SSB Health Services can take up the task of *Rural Sanitation* in a composite manner.

*On the Indo Nepal Border the border population can be taken care of by the SSB personnel & Para Medical Staff to train them in Birth Control clinics &methods thereof, AIDS prevention and other health hazards of national importance. Complacency in tackling such problems can lead to further disaster in managing the health problems. Provision for distribution of free condoms to the SSB personnel and the border population can go a long way in completing this task to a satisfactory level.

*SSB Medical services can play an active role to implement National Immunization Programme (NIS) in the border population especially on INB & IBB not only by the Para Medical Staff, but the local population can also be involved to cater to it. Presently Pulse Polio Immunization Programme (PPIP) is actively supervised by the Sashastra Seema Bal Medical Service:

* Planning for Iodized salt can be taken over by the Sashastra Seema Bal Para Medical staff in their area of operation thereby helping achieve bringing down the national incidence below 10 percent by the year 2010.

*Action plan required especially in the foothills of Sikkim, Darjeeling in West Bengal, Bihar, U.P, UttaraKhand on IndoNepal Border and on Indo Bhutan Border – Assam foothills which are quite prone to mosquito menace and therefore malaria.

*SSBHS can participate in community related Filarial Control programme.

* In the SSB set up where most of the time potable drinking water is not available especially on the Indo Nepal Border, DIARRHOEAL TREATMENT UNITS (DTU) are the order of the day and it should be recognized as important.

*The CPMF personnel are bound by duty to remain out from their family members for months together. Physical requirements being a natural phenomenon for all -as such chances of STD are quite prevalent which requires a long term counseling through VCCT centers- to nullify it.

SSB health services can be utilized quite competently to quash and nullify the effects of the same.

* As far as management and administration is concerned Assured Career Progression of both medical and Para Medical staff should be given due importance.

> * Co- ordination and co-operation between staff of SSBHS & SHS should be another priority area.
>
> * Frequent transfer/postings should be avoided or based on some rationale.

* Proper security for medical personnel especially while working in bordering areas from cordon & search & shelling is a most.

* Another aspect that should be looked into is related with even distribution of job functions.

* Partially skilled and unskilled staff that is present in a large number should be retained.

* Automation is required for technical and economic reasons.

* The Marketing or Publicity requires research and development along with retraining and trimming at the corners.

Keeping in view the SSB philosophy, the recommendations for EFFECTIVE HEALTH SERVICES-A STUDY FOR SASHASTRA SEEMA BAL can lead towards health for all in the years to come.

6.5 CONTRIBUTIONS

The thesis deals with the study of SSBHS of the CPMFs especially on the Indo Nepal Border which has a plethora of fast changing landscapes and situation. The purpose was to plan a Strategy for the Health Services of SSB on the INB. The state of the art Strategic Plan as applicable to the health sector hitherto not studied in proper perspective was taken into consideration. The literature related with it was found to be scanty.

The following are the contributions of this research:

> **Quality Health Care and Infrastructure Development**: Increase safety & quality, affordability and accessibility of health care, including behavioral health care and long term care.

- **Health Promotion and protection, prevention of disease and Prepare for any contingency/Emergency:** Prevent and control disease, injury, illness and disability across the life span, and protect the SSB Personnel/public (5 Kms from the border) from infectious, occupational, environmental disease and terrorist attacks.

- **Service to Mankind through WARB (Welfare and Rehabilitation Board):** Promotion of economic and social well-being of SSB personnel, individuals, families & communities.

- **Research and development with increasing management practices:** Enhance research and development related to health and human services on the INB.

- **Market Share Building:** Via: Minor & Major Medical Civic Actions.

- **Medical:** Augment existing hospital facilities, CME (cont. Medical education), training & practice sessions (for clinical & pm staff) besides provisions for potable drinking water to eradicate gastro- enteritis & related disease for SSB on INB as well as bordering population.

- **Management & Administrative: Management & Administrative reforms in the form of** assured career progression, co-ordination between staff of SSBHS & SHS besides retrainining of staff and computerisation has already been implemented based on the recommendations of the plan and it continues to develop being a continuous process.

- **Publicity (Marketing): The Publicity wing has been revamped to showcase the** HEALTH FOR ALL aspect besides research and development of Photoshop and training of staff.

Although, these are the very essence of our contributions to the field of SSBHS it is submitted that they are not exhaustive. In terms of finality in refinement of our postulates and propositions, further studies are necessary to advance the frontier of knowledge in the field for the betterment of the SSB health services.

6.6 LIMITATIONS

A. The limitations of this research with respect to the SSBHS include:

❖ Understanding the relationship of SSBHS with other CPMFs which is a separate study altogether.

❖ This study also does not specifically address the security of the organization. Security and contingency planning often go hand-in-hand in organizations. Many security features such as fences, controlled access systems, cameras, etc. are taken into consideration when doing contingency planning. However, the security field, which is technologically complex, is beyond the scope of the present study.

❖ Determination of the desirable effects of CME on behavioral outcomes might change SSBHS itself'.

❖ Expanding SSBHS measures to a wider range of age groups as well as on IBB to better understand its developmental course.

B.   This study does not specifically address the information technology (IT) aspects of contingency planning due to the complexity and emergent nature of information systems products. IT departments may have very detailed plans in place to recover hardware, software, telecommunication and other systems. These preparations are usually known as *disaster recovery plans*. It is incumbent upon business continuity personnel, however, to ensure that their IT departments are fully aware of critical systems and recovery priorities. Without the three-prong approach of emergency management, business continuity and disaster recovery, organizational recovery may be severely impeded.

C.   The study also does not consider the problems faced by the other Frontiers who have their own health related problems and are specific for that area. It will require further thrust to study these limitations for the betterment of Jawans and their family members living in these area.

D.   The problems faced by the dependent relations of the SSB jawans serving on the border away from their kith and kin has not been studied in depth which requires thinking and thorough research. A relationship of commonalities of emotional levels of the parent and child needs redefining.

E.   Role and qualifications of instructors needs to be worked on to produce better trained paramedics and other staff. .

6.7 SCOPE FOR FURTHERANCE OF RESEARCH

Many of the identified gaps envisioned for the SSBHS directly impact the personnel. If the project is not funded, there is a greater chance that employees or visitors may suffer injuries or death if a health crisis occurs.

The SSBHS does not have a regular evacuation drill or consistent training material to help employees prepare for disaster at work or home. Our first responders have not been trained in search and rescue and do not have personal protective gear for hazardous material calls. The CPMFs contain numerous chemicals and responder lives can be jeopardized.

Planners are isolated and not sharing knowledge. This situation leaves the SSBHS vulnerable if a planner leaves or is unable to work. Also, in the event of a major disaster, emergency planner's mutual aid will be invaluable.

Examination of the INB hazards, response capabilities and infrastructure were additional issues that might affect SSBHS. It was found that aging infrastructure, regular migration across the border are issues of major concern. Based on various scenarios, the SSBHS could be heavily impacted by the porosity on the border. This warrants further review to determine options. This study does not address the information technology (IT) aspects of the Health services due to the complexity and emerging nature of information systems products.

IT departments may have very detailed plans in place to recover hardware, software, telecommunication and other systems even in the field of health services planning. These preparations are usually known as *disaster recovery plans*. It is incumbent upon the SSB administration, however, to ensure that their IT departments are fully aware of critical systems and recovery priorities. The three-pronged approach of emergency management, business continuity and disaster recovery, recovery of an organizational can be severely curtailed.

This study also does not specifically address the security of the SSBHS in the organization. Security and contingency planning often go hand-in-hand in organizations. Many security features such as fences, controlled access systems, cameras, etc. are taken into consideration when doing contingency planning. This security field, because of its complexities technically, is beyond the scope of the present study involving the SSB Health services.

REFERENCES

1. WHO, AIDS, Image of the Epidemics , Health Situation in the South-East Asia Region Regional office for SEAR, New Delhi. (1994).

2. Indian Management (Vol. 36, No.8), Measurement of Levels of Health, WHO Reg.Publ.Euro, Ser.No.7, P.199. (1997).

3. WHO. Global Health Situations & Projections (1992).

4. Govt. of India. Annual Report, 1984-85, Ministry of Health & Family Welfare (1985).

5. Statistical Outline of India, T.S.L. Deptt. Of Economic & Statistics (1992-93).

6. Cipllo, C.M. The Economic History of World Population, a Pelican Original (1974).

7. Indian Society of Health Administration, Proceedings of the 10th Annual Conference (1990).

8. Oxford University Press. World Bank World Development Report-(1987),

9. CMC Vellore. International Consultation, (Jan, 1991).

10. Baldev Raj & Prasad, B.G. Geriatrics, 25, 142-158 (1970),

11. Griffin C.C. Health Care in Asia- The World Bank, Washington D.C. (1992).

12. Chatterjee, Meera. Indian Women: Their Health & Productivity. World Bank Discussion, paper 109. Washington, D.C. (1990).

13. Zachariah K.C. World Population Projections 1987-88. Edition: Short and long Term Estimates. Baltimore, Md. Johns Hopkins University Press (1988).

14. Heinz Weihrich, "The Tows Matrix: A Tool for Situational Analysis. " Long Range Planning – Pg. 60. (1982)

15. Susanna E. Krentz & Pilskaln S.M. – "Product life cycle – A valid Framework for Business Planning" – Pg-43. (1988) P/143

16. Oxford University Press. UNICEF, The State of the World's Children, - (1987)

17. Banerjee, Meera-Developing Communication Skills – BITS, Pilani, Rajasthan. (1994).

18. Jean Dreze & Amartza Sen. India – Economic Development and Social Opportunity –Osford University Press, (1996).

19. Kerr L. White Health Services Research - An Anthology, Pan American Health Organization (WHO), (1990)

20. German, P.S., Fried, L.P., Annual Review of Public Health Vol. 10. Pg.-325. (1989)

21. Govt. of India, health Information of India DGHS, New Delhi. (1992)

22. Bryson J.M. Strategic Planning for Public & Non Profit Organizations', (1990).

23. David W. Dunlop, Martins J.M. An International Assessment of Health Care Financing, (1982).

24. Griffin, C.C. WHO. Global Health Situations & Projections. (1997)

25. T.S.L. Deptt. Of Economic & Statistics Statistical Outline of India (1992-93)

26. German, P.S., Fried, L.P., Annual Review of Public Health Vol. 10. Pg. -325(1989)

27. Preker A.S., Mckee, M. Mitchtll A. and Wilbul S. Pol Prasart. Strategic management of clinical services 07; 1-14. (2008)

28. Dr. George J. & Srivastava S. HIPA, - Action Research & Planning for Decentralisation. (April 1996).

29. SEARO.N. WHO - Iodine deficiency dissectors . Paper No. 10,N. Delhi(1977)

30. Government of India, Annual Report, DGHC, N. Delhi (1992-93).

31. Clugston, G.A. & Bogchi K. world health forum 7:33 (1986)

32. Govt. of India. Centre calling Nov.1987.,Role of Medical Officer of PHC in Malaria Control, Mass Mailing Unit,MHFW,GOI.(1977).

33. Govt. of India, Bulletin of Rural health statistics in India, DGHC, N. Delhi (June 1993).

34. BASU, R.N. & KAUL, S.M .J.com. Dis, 17(2)131(1985).

35. Sehgal, P.N. J.com.Dis, 19(1)25 et 01(1987)

36. Hopkins, DR. Lanect, 1:96:97. (1985).

37. NICD. Guinea worm eradication programme in India, Revised edition. (1985),

38. Duke, B.O.L. (1985), World health, (March 1984).

39. Nutrition foundation of India .The national Goitre control programme, New Delhi (1983).

40. Govt. of India. National AIDS control programme India, country scenario up date, NACO, M of H&FW N. Delhi. (1987),

41. Govt. of India, Annual report MOH & FW, New Delhi (1993-94).

42. Govt. of India, Ministry of Health & family welfare (1987). Annual report ,(1986-87).

43. Sharma, G.K. & M. Narasimham K.K. L. T.com.Dis 19(1)31. (1987)

44. Govt. of India. Operation manual for malaria action programme (MAP), NMEP, Ministry of health & Family welfare, New Delhi. (1995),

45. Govt. of India Annual report 1995-1996, Ministry of health & family welfare, New Delhi. (1996),

46. WHO Technical report , No. 702 (1984).

47. RAO, C.K. Ind.T.Lep, 59(2)203. (1987)

48. Park, K. Health programmes in India PSM 15,303. (1997),

49. Gupta S.P. T.com. Dis, 17 (2)146. (1985).

50. Govt. of India. Swarth Hind 30(8)177-182. (1986)

51. Catterall R.D. & Nicol C.S. (eds.) Academic press. WHO. Control of sexually transmitted diseases, (1985).

52. Govt. of India   Health information of India 1986, Central Bureau of health Intelligence, DGHS, New Delhi. (1986)

53. Restructuring of Medical set up; GOI, MHA, No. 27012/33/2003/PF f-III9ii), 1st (Sept 2004).

54. Infrastructure Development, Composite Hospital set up, MOF, IFA, Dy. No. 1938/Fin-III/04, (15.09.04).

55. Sector wise staff strength, under Frontier Hqr SSB, Patna, GOI,27012-18/33/35/N.B.-2nd (Sept.2004).

56. Frontier strength Para Medical Staff SSB, Patna, IFA, MHA, Dy. No. 1682/Fin-III/04, (12.08.04).

57. Drug low enforcement Trig. Vol-I page 1 to 6; NCB, India,(2005)

58. Drug low enforcement Trg. Vol-I page 42-46, NCB-India,(2005)

59. Mc Ardle, Catch & Katch. 2001; National heart, Lungs & Blood Institute, physiological Assessment of human fitness, E-186. (1998)

LIST OF PUBLICATIONS OF CANDIDATE

During the study on **"A Strategic Plan for Effective Health Services – A Study for Sashastra Seema Bal"** different papers were published/presented at different forums and incorporated in the SSB for the benefit of jawans and their family members.

A few of them are mentioned below –

1. **Guillain Barre Syndrome** – A paper presented at all India Doctors Conference duly attended by more than 50 Doctors and Peer reviewed by Masters in their field. The Director General-SSB and other prominent personalities from SSB and outside the ambit of SSB thoroughly enjoyed the presentation.

   It was commended as the best presentation and the recommendations have already been implemented in the CPMFs namely SSB and others in this regard.

2. **A pictorial presentation of flood relief carried out by different units under the Aegis of Frontier Hqrs. SSB, Patna**- The flood relief work that was carried out during the devastating floods in Bihar especially on the Indo-Nepal border near Birpur was a cause for concern and action was taken to stop the annihilation being caused by the Kosi.

   The whole work was seen by a panel of senior dignitaries which included the Inspector General, the Dy.Inspector General, Commandants besides the Director General and later the work was sent to the Home Ministry for their perusal.

This is a regular feature in this region every year leading to severe Gastro-Enteritis, Diarrhoea & Dysentry, Typhoid, Kala-Azar & other Water Borne Disease.

The Preventive aspects that have been propounded & recommended have already been implemented for the betterment of the SSB Jawans and their family members.

3. Sashastra Seema Bal – The First to Reach.-A write up on the devastation caused during the 2008 floods near Birpur on INB where the SSB is deployed.

    To tackle such problems action oriented recommendations have been propounded and implementation is on the cards especially in the future.

4. **Tackling Terror – A Formidable Challenge for Police in India**. A write-up on how to combat terrorism and tackling terror in the aftermath of a terrorist attack and why it happens is the main concern of this article. It represented the Frontier Headquarter-SSB-Patna for the PMs Gold Cup competition which has been well appreciated by the officers concerned.

    The fight between haves & have-nots is the crux of the problem which has to be controlled to come to a semblance of sanity and providing employment /business opportunity to the also rans.

    Action has already been started in this regard by the central Govt. in the form of NREGA & PMGSY & NRHM.

5. Article in News Profile-[In English on Sports]-"National Himalayan Trekking Expedition".

6. Article in Prabhat Khabar (Eng.) - English cricket-On Fraternity vacation.

7. Article in N.M.O. – AIDS- A Global Problem. Few   other articles   have also been well appreciated in this regard and ***recommendations have been applied through NACO & SSB VCCT centers.***

8. Article at M.G.M.C.H. - From Panic to Mastery- and what's in between.

9. Article in News-Profile-[In English on Medicine] –All articles recommendations have been utilized at different forums and SSBHS is also aware or them and acts accordingly.

    a) Battling Diabetes- The easy way.

    b) Cholera-Dos & Don'ts.

    c) A Heart to Heart talk about Heart.

    d) Aismoc'92- An overview.

    e) Obesity- you can over come it.

    f) Filaria- a curse to humanity

    g) Diabetes Mellitus – An update.

10. Diabetes, Obesity, Hypertension & Drug Abuse is quite prevalent in the department. Recommendations on them are utilized for the SSB personnel at all levels.

These are a few samples of papers /articles presented/ published down the years at different forums. It is a sample of a few such and not exhaustive. However work on Hepatitis –B and Kala-Azar is still going on because of their prevalence in the population at large and SSB personnel on the INB. These two require further research in the years to come.

BIOGRAPHY OF SUPERVISOR

1. Name : Dr. C.R. Roy

2. Present Designation, : Consultant Patho/physiology,
   Official: J.B. Poly Clinic Address
   Email Address Telephone No. and Sushrut Nagar,
   P.O- Sushrut Nagar, Near N.B.
   Medical College and Hospital,
   Dist: Darjeeling
   (W.B.) T/No. 0353-2585398.
   Email- drcrroy@yahoo.co.uk.

3. Permanent Address : As above.

4. Date of Birth : 1st Feb. 1933.

5. Educational Qualification : Matric – 1949 – 2nd Div.

   Sc. - 1952 – 2nd Div.

   B.Sc. - 1954 – 2nd Div.

   M.Sc. - 1959 – 2nd Div.

   Ph. D. - 1968 – Very Good

6. Academic Distinctions attained:

7. Professional Career beyond Master's Degree to present date in chronological order-

   a) Reader and HOD Physiology - N.B. Medical College & Hospital.

   b) Consultant Patho/Physiologist - J.B. Poly Clinic, Susrut Nagar

8. Board field of research interests with specific areas of involvement -

    a)   Bio-Chemistry

    b)   Physiology

9. Publications; Studies on Blood and nutritional physiology, and others

10. Type of industrial and consultancy work done- Hospital like Army, SSB, BSF, Tea Garden Hospital, Poly Clinics etc.

11. Patents obtained

12. Visits abroad and nature of assignment

13. Membership of professional societies – Indian Science Congress.

14. Doctoral degrees thesis already supervised – Dr. Bikash Ghosh – Problems of nutrition Nutrition in Himul.

15. Number of Ph. D Candidates – Currently registered – 01.

16. State in what manner connected with candidate's organization and proposed place of   work- Consultancy Work relative with Patho/Physiology, Haematology, Echo Cardio   graphy   and Radio Diagnosis.

LIST OF APPENDICES

SSB HOSPITAL

22ND BN.SSB, RANIDANGA

Doctor's Orders

Patients Name :   Age: Sex :   Consultant :

Date	Clinical Findings	Medicines & Treatment	Investigations

		225	

COMPOSITE HOSPITAL, SSB, PURNEA

OP NO. :   IP NO. :   Service wards

Note if :

                                    Medico legal :

Patient's Name   Age

Father's /Husband Name   Sex

                                            Religion
                                            Occupation
                                            Blood Group

DOA : Time: DOD : Time:

Referred by :

Allergic to

Diagnosis   Provisional

                   FinalConsultant:

Case Summary (To be filled on discharge)

Condition on discharge Cured Relieved Referred LAMA Expired

Authorization:

Permission is hereby given for the performance of any form of treatment essential for the case of my patient including any diagnostic examination, biopsy, transfusion, operation and administration of any anesthesia as may be deemed advisable in the course of hospital admission. The risk of various procedures has been explained to me and I am willing to undertake the risk.

Name   Relationship   Sign

Operation Request

It has been explained to me that I am suffering from ....
....
.... and after all the necessary examination/ investigation that
.... is the treatment for the same.

I request that I/my relative (Name & relationship) may have/has
.... (Procedure done as a cure for
my/his/her illness.

I have no objection to using ....
Anesthesia is expected that the doctors performing this operation will be
.... But in unforeseen circumstances this may change.

I give the doctors permission to take whatever steps they think necessary
should something unexpected arise.

I do not give permission for ....
....

(Not above anything you specifically refuse to allow)

Understand that I may discuss this with a relative or friend before signing
this form.

Signed: Date:

Witness:

SSB HOSPITAL

COMPOSITE HOSPITAL PURNEA

DISCHARGE NOTE

Name of Patient   :

Age/Sex   :

Address   :

Date of Admission :   IP NO. :

Date of Discharge :   OP NO.:

Complaints   :

Investigations   :

Diagnosis   :